Praise for *Full-Filled*

"Written with great warmth, wit, and insight, this book offers a realistic way to let go of unhealthy eating habits by giving yourself the nurturing and compassion you actually crave."

—Kristin Neff, Ph.D., author of *Self-Compassion: Stop Beating Yourself Up and Leave Insecurity Behind*

"Renee Stephens has written a reliable companion to take with you on your weight loss journey. The guidance it offers in Chapter 3 alone could change your relationship with food and your body forever. Do yourself a favor and stop any ridiculous diet you may currently be on and buy this book. And then, don't just read it. Do it. If you do, you can expect to find a permanent solution to the struggle, not just another temporary fix. An important read for anyone wanting to lose weight."

—Brooke Castillo, author of *If I Am So Smart, Why Can't I Lose Weight?*

Praise for Renée Stephens

"Renee, I thank you over and over each day!"

—Joy Holloway-D'avilar, New Jersey

"I was a normal healthy little girl, but someone mentioned me getting 'pudgy' (as many children do right before they take a growth spurt), and that was it. I've been fat ever since . . . off and on. Thank you for saying everything I've needed to hear and never knew where to find it . . . Thank you thank you thank you. You are saving my sanity!"

—Jayme Stephens, Arkansas

Full❋Filled

The 6-Week Weight Loss Plan for Changing
Your Relationship with Food
—and Your Life—
from the Inside Out

Renée Stephens

with Samantha Rose

Free Press

New York   London   Toronto   Sydney   New Delhi

Free Press
A Division of Simon & Schuster, Inc.
1230 Avenue of the Americas
New York, NY 10020

Copyright © 2011 by Renée Stephens and Samantha Rose

All rights reserved, including the right to reproduce this book or portions thereof in any form whatsoever. For information address Free Press Subsidiary Rights Department, 1230 Avenue of the Americas, New York, NY 10020

First Free Press hardcover edition January 2012

FREE PRESS and colophon are trademarks of Simon & Schuster, Inc.

For information about special discounts for bulk purchases, please contact Simon & Schuster Special Sales at 1-866-506-1949 or business@simonandschuster.com.

The Simon & Schuster Speakers Bureau can bring authors to your live event. For more information or to book an event contact the Simon & Schuster Speakers Bureau at 1-866-248-3049 or visit our website at www.simonspeakers.com.

Designed by Ruth Lee-Mui

Manufactured in the United States of America

1   3   5   7   9   10   8   6   4   2

Library of Congress Cataloging-in-Publication Data
Stephens, Renée.
Full-filled : the 6-week weight-loss plan for changing your relationship with food—and your life—from the inside out / Renée Stephens with Samantha Rose.—1st ed.
        p.   cm.
Includes index.
1. Weight loss—Psychological aspects. I. Rose, Samantha. II. Title.
        RM222.2.S776 2011
    613.2'5—dc23   2011029232

ISBN 978-1-4516-4122-6
ISBN 978-1-4516-4123-3 (ebook)

To all those who still struggle.
May you know that the change you desire,
or something even better,
is possible for you.

Contents

Full ✳ Filled

Introduction

Let me guess. You're fed up with low fat, no fat, calorie counting, carb control, and one failed weight loss attempt after another. Along with other dieters, you reject the tired mentality of extreme deprivation and control in a food plan. And you're ready to embrace the radical-new weight loss approach of *Full-Filled*, one that millions of others who were fed up like you have successfully benefited from. You will drop excess physical pounds on this program, but you will first get to the root of why you eat and lose your "spiritual" weight.

You see, your weight struggle and your overall sense of happiness and personal fulfillment really have little to do with food. This realization has opened the eyes of countless men and women who were desperate to break their cycle of overeating once and for all—and it helped them succeed.

Weight loss is a spiritual practice. Who knew?

It's true: your struggle with food relates to deeply personal and spiritual issues that go far beyond what you ordered for lunch. Yet there's a little more to losing weight than this single realization. Getting to the root of your weight struggle and identifying why you eat the way you do is just the first step towards taking off the pounds in a reliable, lasting way. To permanently lose the weight you've spent so many frustrating years lugging around, you need the transformative program laid out in this book. The Full-Filled program will identify and also heal your underlying food issues, and it will provide you with the specific tools to create new, healthful habits that will make you slim and healthy for a lifetime.

And I will help you do all that.

My name is Renée Stephens, and I'm a leading diet and weight loss coach. I'm also a former food addict. I understand all too well how painful and exhausting the weight struggle can be. I spent more years than I'd like to admit (okay, twenty) consumed by my food addiction and punishing myself over my imperfect body. Then I discovered the secret of freedom that I share with you in the pages of this book. Inspired by my own battle with food and body image, I've synthesized some of the world's most advanced mind and behavior-changing techniques to create an easy, intuitive step-by-step weight loss program. *Full-Filled* will permanently change how you think about and behave around food so that you can finally have the body and the life you've always desired.

You see, whether you're 5 or 15 or 150 pounds heavier than you'd like to be, understand that your weight didn't land on your body accidentally. It's there for a reason. Whether you realize it or not, that heaping bowl of pasta you like to eat is satisfying more than your taste buds. Maybe it provides a quick hit of relief from boredom, frustration, loneliness, or grief. It may be that food gives you a sense of comfort and protection, or perhaps you simply consider that extra mouthful a well-deserved treat after a long day of toil and sacrifice. Whatever your reasons for eating and overeating certain foods, in order for you to enjoy significant and lasting weight loss, you have to identify *why* you eat the way you do and find better ways to satisfy your true hunger, without food.

You might be thinking, "Yeah, right. And how many years of therapy will that take?" The good news is that changing how you think and thus what you crave and how you behave is quicker and easier than you ever dreamed possible when you have the right tools. You can "rewire" your mind to think differently. And since all behavior begins with a thought, when you change your mind about food, you change your behavior around food.

In the pages that follow, I will give those powerful tools to you and teach you how to use them as you hear about other people's personal success stories. You'll finish this journey with a whole bag of transformative tips and tricks that have progress built right into them. Not only will they set you up for significant weight loss and the no-fail techniques for keeping it off permanently, they'll help you discover:

1. What you're getting out of overeating (hint: it's something positive)
2. How to pinpoint the foods and situations that automatically trigger you to go overboard
3. Why your big-time "screwups" are actually essential to your success
4. How to think like and become a slim and healthy person, no matter how long you've fought the battle of the bulge
5. How weight loss can open the door to even greater rewards in your life

Surprisingly, even though this is a weight loss program, I will spend very little time talking about what you should or shouldn't put in your mouth. Nor will I tell you definitively when and how much to eat. Yes, I'll share with you the foods that will make weight loss happen faster and easier, and I'll even throw in a few of my favorite recipes, but for the most part, we will put food to the side.

Instead, you'll focus on sparking a powerful transformation that will leave you satisfied on the inside and slim and healthy on the outside. I call this "losing weight from the inside out," and once you start thinking and behaving in this new way, you'll soon discover that losing weight is actually quite easy, and even pleasurable.

It may sound too good to be true, but let me assure you, it's for real—and you can do it. With more than 3.5 million downloads to date, my *Inside Out Weight Loss* audio podcast, based on the principle that weight loss has to be easy and enjoyable to last a lifetime, is the number one weight loss podcast on iTunes. I've consulted for Weight Watchers International as a behavioral weight loss expert, and I've run seminars and programs about weight loss for Fortune 500 companies, including Whole Foods, Gap, and Oracle. I'm also a featured teacher in *The Inner Weigh*, a documentary film that introduces viewers to the idea that permanent weight loss begins within.

I work with both men and women who have spent years trying to free themselves from their weight struggle and regain control of their lives. They include the perpetually overweight who believe their metabolism is to blame, binge eaters who can barely get through breakfast without overeating, bulimics who hide their secret from family and friends, and failed dieters who spend the majority of their days thinking about what not to eat or suffering from guilt over what they did eat and who believe that no matter how hard they try, they're destined to be at war with food and their bodies. Each of them had tried everything from fad diets to psychotherapy and twelve-step programs. Nothing worked for them until they found my program, now available for the first time in its complete form here in *Full-Filled*.

As my clients and listeners discover along the way, losing weight can actually be a door to even larger rewards in other areas of your life. I hope you will discover this, too. Of course, our first order of business is weight loss, but my ultimate goal is to help you understand that ending the weight struggle isn't simply about dropping a few pounds for your high school reunion or a swimsuit vacation. It's about turning your old mind-set inside out and waking up to the rest of your life.

Think about it. How much time have you spent obsessing over your weight? How many days, weeks, or years have you beat yourself up, convinced that because of how you look, you aren't "good enough"? If you're like me, you've spent much of your life struggling with yourself in this way. What do you think happens when all that mental and emotional energy is released and returned back to you?

I'll tell you exactly what happens. You start discovering passions you didn't realize you had. You start showing up fully to your family and loved ones. You start finding satisfaction outside food, and ultimately, as you forgive and accept yourself as you are, you create a life that you truly love. Those are big promises for a weight loss program. But trust me: on this, I speak from experience.

My Story

My own weight struggle began when I was eleven years old. My best girlfriend and I decided to go on a diet because both our mothers were big-time dieters. In fact, one of my earliest memories of Mom is of her filling out the Weight Watchers chart on the refrigerator door. Like our mothers and all their girlfriends, we learned how to count calories and obsess about everything we ate. By the age of thirteen, I'd perfected food deprivation (starving), bingeing (eating way past full in an uncontrollable frenzy), and atoning (by starving myself or exercising to exhaustion).

As a binger, I'd go on late-night rampages, stuffing myself with whatever I could find, from cupcakes to chocolate syrup, from cheese and crackers to butter on cheese and crackers! I ate from the trash can, I ate from the freezer, and I always ate in secret. Disgusted with myself, I'd retreat to my bedroom to face the pictures of models I'd taped to my walls, horrified that I'd just pushed myself further away from reaching my picture-perfect ideal. In despair, I'd jump up and down for hours at a time in an attempt to burn off the calories, then starve myself for days, until I'd break down and begin the cycle of overeating all over again.

By the time I turned nineteen, my eating habits and remedies had spun completely out of control. I'd tried every fad diet out there, from liquid protein fasts to grapefruit-and-egg plateau busters to the Scarsdale and Cambridge diets and even a supervised weight loss program where I was allowed only 750 calories a day. (My "safe" foods at the time included "protein crunchies," which look not unlike gerbil food.) The results were always the same: quick weight loss, complete with the proclamation that I'd never, ever go back to my old ways, followed by uncontrolled eating and boomerang weight gain. As I went up and down the scale, I mercilessly beat myself up for lacking the strength and sheer will necessary to permanently drop the pounds.

My eating issues continued into my twenties, when I finally mustered up the courage to consult a nutritionist. She asked me to keep a food diary, and for weeks, I honestly reported what I ate. When my nutritionist reviewed my entries, she wrote the following note on my chart: "Frequent use of chocolate syrup." Embarrassing but true. My favorite indulgence was chocolate from a squeeze-top bottle. She told me I was a compulsive eater and referred me to Overeaters Anonymous (OA), a twelve-step program based on the principles of Alcoholics Anonymous.

After joining OA and getting to know others in the program, I realized that I wasn't the only person on the planet plagued by food guilt and uncontrollable eating and that the reason I ate wasn't that I was crazy. I faithfully followed the OA program for three years and successfully lost more than 30 pounds and four clothing sizes. (On my small frame, this amount of weight loss seemed huge to me, mainly because of how much I'd built up my weight issue in my mind over the years.)

I clearly remember the day when I reached my magic number on the scale—a day I'd always hoped for and dreamed of. My friends in OA were so proud of me. Yet I still felt unhappy. I'd always thought that if I were slimmer, people would like me more, I'd have a fabulous relationship, I'd advance in my career, and I'd be happy. How wrong I was. Even though I'd reached my "ideal" weight, I was still depressed.

Overeaters Anonymous helped me understand that my eating habits were somehow linked to my emotional life, but I failed to make a clear connection. Still nagged by beliefs of my own unworthiness and convinced that my true nature was somehow flawed, I remained imprisoned, locked into thinking that I'd always be a binge eater and would backslide if I didn't watch myself. Years after leaving the program, I continued to obsessively weigh and measure everything I ate and critically scrutinize myself in front of the mirror.

I tortured myself well into my thirties, gaining a reputation among friends and coworkers as "high maintenance" and weird around food. Gluten-free, yeast-free, fat-free—I was a waiter's worst nightmare! Afraid I'd return to my old ways in a moment of weakness, I desperately clung to control. Finally, at age thirty-five, exhausted and stressed-out by my relentless struggle, my body went on strike and shut down. I was diagnosed with chronic fatigue syndrome, and it was that flat-on-my-back, debilitated state that finally allowed me to understand that my weight issue was directly tied to how I was living my life. I'd dedicated fifteen years to a career that I didn't enjoy in high-tech marketing and international business, a professional goal I'd set for myself based on what I thought others expected me to do.

After years of chasing the wrong dream for the wrong reasons, my body and spirit had had it. Despite having lost more than 30 pounds through OA, I'd continued to be a freak around food because I'd never dealt with my real hunger—which was to be accepted and loved for who I was. For as long as I could remember, I'd used food to stuff down feelings of inadequacy and to fuel my relentless push to be someone worthy of love, acceptance, even employment. I'd spent an outrageous amount of energy trying to prove myself to the world, afraid that, if I dropped my disguise, I'd be seen for who I really was—a woman not thin enough, fit enough, smart enough, pretty enough. A woman not worthy of being loved! I finally realized that I couldn't go on pretending to be anyone other than who I was; my body wouldn't let me. So I was forced to just be me.

But who was the real Renée? I wasn't sure, but I was determined to figure it out. I quit my six-figure job at IBM with only a loose plan to pursue new interests. I'd always been fascinated by human motivation, so I began researching the motivation of the mind. I studied neurolinguistic programming (NLP), which allowed me to understand how motivation works. I then discovered the work of Dr. Robert Dee McDonald, the developer of the Destination Method, which is a holistic approach to NLP that works with body, mind, and spirit. I discovered that if I applied what I was learning about the power of motivation to my own food issues, I got results I didn't even know were possible. For the first time in my life, I began to experience freedom and ease around both food and my body. Soon my classmates were asking me to help them, too.

By synthesizing the tools that most helped me—neuroscience, hypnotherapy, and life coaching that goes hand in hand with sound nutritional guidelines—I developed a powerful program for overcoming overeating and negative body image. I started a private practice and began speaking and running programs for companies. In 2007, I started my *Inside Out Weight Loss* podcast, giving listeners a place to "plug into" my program for thirty-minute jolts of motivation for reliable, long-lasting change. And now I've written *Full-Filled,* the book that pulls my program together all in one place—in an easy, step-by-step format that takes you from tortured to trim.

My inside-out weight loss approach not only dramatically changed the course of my personal and professional life, it has inspired countless men and women to end their internal struggle, too. They've found slimmer and healthier bodies, fulfillment, longevity, and an awakening to the rest of their lives.

And guess what? You're next.

I am thrilled to be your guide.

Love,
Renée Stephens

How the Full-Filled Program Works

To get the results you've spent so many years desperately fighting for, I encourage you to fully immerse yourself in this program for the next six weeks. Jump right in, and give it everything you've got. I mean it—*everything*. The tools in this program are extraordinarily effective, and they work faster than any others I know of to get you the body and life you desire. But they work only if you use them. Over the course of the next six weeks, apply them to every situation you can in your life.

This may sound like a heavy-duty commitment, but now consider how much time and energy you've spent struggling with your weight over the years. Six weeks is nothing, right? Once you've made the initial investment of getting set up and charged up about permanent, reliable weight loss, I'll ask only that you spend about ten minutes a day fine-tuning your progress.

How easy is that? You've been on diets that have demanded much more, I'm sure. All I ask is that you open your mind to a new way of thinking and that you put your health and happiness at the top of your priority list. If you can do that, you'll be well on your way to permanently transforming your relationship with food, your body, and yourself in a month and a half. In fact, substantial changes, even dramatic ones, might happen sooner than that.

The Full-Filled program is divided into six weeks, or cycles, of continuous progress. Subtle changes begin happening quickly and immediately, and the long-term benefits extend far beyond the pages of this book. From the very first day of the Full-Filled program (that's today!), you'll begin to think in a completely different way that will, ideally and more than likely, inspire you to change how you eat and live forevermore. In that respect, the progress you will make over the next six weeks is limitless. Furthermore, your progress along the way will become the basis for your long-term maintenance.

Most diet and weight loss programs save maintenance for the end, when your willpower is all but exhausted. Some don't even provide a long-term plan, naively assuming that you will stay on the diet forever.

The Full-Filled program is different. I address the maintenance piece of the program up front, because if you finally lose the excess weight you've been carrying around for so many frustrating years and have no realistic plan for keeping it off, what's the point of losing it in the first place? On the Full-Filled program, long-term motivation and maintenance are built in from day one. You may find that at the end of the six weeks, you're exactly where you want to be. Or you may find that you want to repeat some key exercises or rework the entire program for additional benefit. However you individualize your experience, the Full-Filled program allows for a continuous cycle of progress and reward.

The Full-Filled Weight-Release Journal

Before you jump in and begin Week 1 of the Full-Filled program, I encourage you to get a journal that you will dedicate to your weight loss journey. Keep it by your side throughout the next six weeks. Your journal can be as plain as a spiral notebook or something more elegant. The simple act of writing your thoughts down as you progress through the program will keep you in the present moment and help you become aware of how you feel from week to week. A written progress report will also keep you accountable for your actions and help you better track your thoughts and eating habits as they change. Clients often tell me that journaling allows them to go deeper into the Full-Filled program and stay focused on their long-term intentions. So even if you're not the journaling type, make note of your insights and progress. You'll be glad you did.

Put In to Get Out

In addition to encouraging you to fully engage and participate in the Full-Filled program from day one, I also invite you to—no, actually I insist that you—seek out or create a support community of family, friends, neighbors, or coworkers who either have been where you are now or are currently where you are now and would like to accompany you on your weight loss journey. Your community could be as small as a party of two—you and your BFF—or a larger group of ten or more. Either way, research proves it: when you enlist outside support, you create for yourself a system of encouragement and accountability, which will dramatically accelerate your progress and keep you on track towards reliable, permanent change.

Reaching out to others with whom you reveal your deepest, darkest eating secrets might be the last thing you want to do. When I was still at war with my weight, sharing the details of my late-night binges felt scary and shameful. I was the superwoman who could accomplish anything alone and quietly if I only applied the right amount of will and determination. Yet hidden underneath all my go-it-alone bravado was fear that others would see how weak and truly weird around food I was. I was absolutely convinced that if they knew the truth, they'd reject me.

That skewed thinking was why letting others in became absolutely key to my progress. I discovered that when I confided in others who similarly understood the weight struggle, they accepted me. They did not judge me harshly when I made admissions such as "I ate out of the trash can last night." That acceptance and non-judgmentalism gave me the superwoman strength and motivation I needed in order to push forward on the days when I felt powerless and incapable of solving my weight problem on my own. As my teacher Dr. Robert McDonald says, "We are wounded in community and healed in community."

So buddy up, open up, and stay connected throughout the next six weeks with people who are positive and kind and who are likely to provide you with valuable encouragement and insight. You'll be glad you did. If you aren't quite ready to reach out and connect with others, no worries. Begin to work through the Full-Filled program on your own as a "warm-up," and when you're ready to ratchet up your progress, share your stories, and receive outside support, you'll know just how to do it in the ways I outline below.

Here are a few ways to build your support group.

Create a Community Offline

Recruit your sister, your best friend from school, your coworker, your neighbor. Ask if they struggle with their weight and tell them you've found a new program that heals your underlying food issues and transforms your current cravings, so that you lose your desire to overeat while you gain an appetite for a more healthful lifestyle. Invite them to get a copy of this book and join you in building a support group. Make a commitment to one another that, no matter what, you will show up, especially when you screw up (which is a big part of the program, by the way). Designate a place to meet or a time to talk on the phone or correspond by e-mail. If you're going to meet, choose a place where you feel safe and comfortable sharing the ups and downs of your weight-release journey.

How you conduct your meetings is entirely up to you, but here are some suggestions to get you going. First and foremost, I recommend that you kick off your meeting time by setting and sharing your intentions for yourself and for the group. Scientists have proved that intentions have the power to set your mind to act towards a desired goal or outcome. Setting intentions is like telling your life where you want it to go. Imagine hopping into a taxi and when the driver asks you, "Where to?" you answer, "Anywhere but here." You wouldn't get very far, would you? To move forward, you must be very clear and specific about where you want to end up.

Setting an intention for every week of the Full-Filled program will give you direction and focus as you work towards a new, slim, and healthy you. It's not quite the same as setting a future goal, because setting your intention begins the process of transformation in the present. By simply stating your intention, you jump-start change *now*. Know, too, that when two or more people set an intention together—a collective intention—it becomes much more powerful. This is why I recommend that each member of your group write out his or her intentions before your meeting and share them aloud with the group.

After you set your intentions, let each member take a turn answering the following questions and receiving support and feedback from the group. If time restrictions are a consideration for your group (if you only have a half hour to meet, for example), ask everyone to write out his or her answers before the meeting.

I encourage you to really dig in when answering these questions. Bring your honesty and your emotions to the meeting. Cry, laugh, and stamp your feet. It will significantly accelerate your progress and bring you and your group closer together.

1. What positive shifts and changes have you noticed in yourself since our last meeting? Be sure to focus on the positive here.

2. What do you want to happen between now and our next meeting? For example, "I want to feel relaxed around food at the party I'm attending and focus on the people instead."

3. How will you know when you have it? For example, "I'll know because when I get home after the party, I'll feel just right in my tummy—neither too full nor too hungry—and renewed by the connections I've made."

4. What's stopping you from having it now? In other words, what's scary about having it?

Create a Community Online

If you can't meet your group members in person, not to worry. Technology lets you connect with people anywhere in the world anytime you wish. Try any of the following methods.

Yahoo! Group

Join an online group you can immediately plug into for valuable support and advice. I have a thriving Inside Out Weight Loss Yahoo! group available through a link on my website at www.insideoutweightloss.com

Note: This is not a collective bellyache group. It's a decidedly positive, upbeat place where you are likely to meet others who, like you, are just starting the program and who are willing and excited to go through the steps with you. This group is a safe place for you to share your experiences, track your progress, and ask for support. It's run by volunteers who are working and living the Full-Filled program.

Private Group

Create a private online group you can immediately plug into for valuable support and advice. Amy, a client of mine, recruited a girlfriend to join her on her weight loss journey. They didn't have time to meet every day or even once a week, so they corresponded through daily e-mails and text messages. By connecting regularly, they were able to support each other every step of the way, sharing their progress, challenges, and breakthroughs. Their partnership played a key role in Amy's ability to lose more than 70 pounds and regain self-confidence and a positive body image.

Conference Calls

Set up a conference call with your support group. You can find a variety of free conference call services by searching for "free conference calls" online. I've made some of my closest friends through virtual mastermind groups, where people with different experiences and ideas hop onto a group line to collaborate with, brainstorm with, and provide support to help others in the group achieve their purpose.

Videoconferencing

Use Skype or a similar program to make free Internet calls using your computer or mobile phone. The built-in webcam on most devices turns a standard call into a videoconference.

Renée Stephens on Facebook

"Like" Renée Stephens on Facebook (facebook.com/reneestephens fanpage) fan, where I regularly post tips and personal stories, and where I encourage my followers to buddy up and support one another.

Renée Stephens on Twitter

Follow me on Twitter (@StephensRenee), where I regularly post motivational thoughts as well as links to supporting articles on the subjects of health, fitness, and weight release, and where you can easily connect with others living the Full-Filled program.

You have many ways to connect and feel supported. Find the method that works best for you and your lifestyle.

Creating Motivation for Lasting Change

How long have you struggled with your weight? Has it been years? Decades? Your whole lifetime? If you are like the majority of the people I work with and help, food and body image are not new challenges for you, but rather struggles that have been weighing you down for much too long. If you've tried every diet out there with no lasting success, you may have asked yourself if anything will help you put a stop to your food issues and forever end your war with your weight.

The work you do in the pages ahead will be very different from anything you've done in the past. The most notable difference is that you will not need to control, restrict, or deprive yourself of food. Instead, you'll set out to change your mind about food. Chances are, you've devoted a lot of time and energy to your current ideas about your body and what goes into it, so adjusting your mind-set will require renewed focus and attention, but I think you'll be pleased at how quickly you'll notice both internal and external changes in yourself. I also think you'll be surprised and delighted at how easy and enjoyable this weight loss program is compared with anything you've tried before.

Associating weight loss with enjoyment may be an idea that's a bit hard for you to swallow, but the two actually go hand in hand. In fact, they must go hand in hand to get positive results. If your weight loss program is easy and enjoyable, it will last a lifetime. If it's hard, it won't work for the long term, which is exactly why "successful" dieters usually aren't successful for long. Generally, within one year, 95 percent of dieters regain the weight they lost. And within five years, a staggering 99 percent are right back where they started.

Not you. This time, you're changing for good.

Before we jump into Week 1 of the Full-Filled program, let me say a few words about the words "weight loss." Loss has a negative association; when we "lose" something, our subconscious mind infers that we've misplaced something we very much wanted to keep around. Our tendency is to immediately set out to find it again. And guess what? Most people who lose weight do indeed find it again! Since I don't think that's your desire here, we need a better term or at least a few alternatives to pick and choose from. Throughout the pages ahead, I will frequently interchange the term "weight loss" with more positive connotations such as "weight release" and "dropping weight."

In Week 1 of the Full-Filled program, you will learn:
- How your present-day reality is the key to jump-starting a fulfilling future
- The importance of "away-from" motivation and "towards" motivation
- How simply dreaming about the life and body you desire will spark big-time behavior change

Where Are You Now, and Why Do You Want to Change?

As you begin Week 1 of the Full-Filled program, **set your intention to create motivation for long-lasting change**. Remember, setting your intention begins the process of transformation in the present. By simply stating your intention, you jump-start change now. Record your intentions in your journal, too. Once your intention to create motivation for long-lasting change is firmly rooted in your mind, take a mental snapshot of yourself today. If you can, stand up from where you're sitting now and go take a long look at yourself in the nearest mirror.

Why do I want you to do this? Your transformation into a slimmer, healthier you begins with assessing exactly where you are now and why you want to change. Taking a mental snapshot of yourself today will not only help you identify the work you want to do over the course of the next six weeks, it will also allow you to fully appreciate the progress you make along the way.

In addition to taking a mental snapshot, consider taking an actual photo of yourself today, and paste it in the front of your weight-release journal. And when you have the photo taken, be sure to look miserable! This is your "before" photo, so let it all hang out. I know, it's not fun. But just imagine how great it will feel to look back at the photo in the near future and appreciate how far you've come.

Food for Thought

As you begin reading this book and set your intention for this journey, take a moment to think of all the others across space and time who are also reading this book and are also on this journey. Like you, they have struggled. Like you, they have hopes and dreams. Send them your compassion and support, your wishes that they, too, will achieve their intentions in the service of their highest good, and feel their support coming back to you, making your journey that much easier every step of the way.

Tracking your progress is an important piece of the Full-Filled program. Imagine for a moment a patch of grass in your front, side, or backyard or in a park near you. If you wanted to grow a garden there, you wouldn't just scatter a packet of seeds and expect them to grow and flourish without first upturning the soil, planting the seeds, and nourishing them with proper tending, light, and water. You need to tend the garden if you want it to grow. Throughout the days and weeks ahead, the new thoughts and habits you will be cultivating are very much like seeds you plant in a garden. In order to thrive, you need to nurture the seeds of change, and one of the ways you will do this is by acknowledging and appreciating the incremental shifts in your mind and body. This awareness will provide you with the energy and motivation you need in order to grow into a new, happier, and healthier you.

Oftentimes, people who struggle with their weight and body image are so used to berating themselves that they rarely notice when the seedlings of new, positive behaviors start to emerge. As a result, the new behaviors don't have a chance to take root and grow. When you don't celebrate your progress, you run the risk of slipping into what I call "success amnesia." That is when a thought or a habit disappears so thoroughly that you forget you ever had it! You even forget that you overcame it. I've seen many clients slip into success amnesia, and though it's not necessarily a problem, it's certainly a missed opportunity to celebrate a win. Think about it: when you recognize that you can overcome something as seemingly entrenched as your issues with weight and body image, you will know that you can handle just about anything life throws at you.

I once had a client who'd gone from regular food and wine binges after a hard day's work to being able to eat and drink moderately—and enjoy it. In a follow-up session together, she shared with me that she was facing a big challenge at work and doubted that she could ever make it through. I said to her, "Well, wait a minute. You've just resolved a lifelong struggle with food and your weight. Don't you think you can handle a little work stress?" She looked at me in surprise and smiled as she realized that of course she could! Then not only did she face her professional challenge head-on, she also later quit her job and launched her own business, something she'd never before thought was possible.

Go ahead and snap that mental picture of where you are today. What do you see? Let me guess. You're not happy with your body, and you want to release weight? That's a given. But what about today's picture do you *specifically* want to change? Let me give you a few examples of what I mean.

Maybe you're someone who eats "good" all day but overeats at dinner and continues to eat even after the dishes are washed and put away. If so, you'd probably like to change that specific nighttime behavior.

Perhaps you're someone who piles your plate high at every meal as if you'll never see another one. If so, you might want to do some work around your idea of what's "enough." And if food, for you, is your number one go-to in stressful times, you likely want to change that method of stress relief.

See where I'm going here? You don't just want to release weight, you want to change the specific behaviors that define your particular weight struggle. Make sense?

Take the next few minutes to dig into the exercise below. You will want to write down your insights in your Full-Filled Weight-Release Journal. Be as brief or as prolific as you'd like. Just write. If you haven't yet dedicated a journal to your weight-release journey, make it a priority this week. Having a written account of your progress will help you track your thoughts and eating habits as they change.

And they *will* change. Many of the Dig In exercises in this book build on one another, so having a written record to refer back to over the next six weeks will be very helpful. Start by documenting your answers to and insights into each of the weekly Dig In exercises. I also encourage you to make a practice of writing daily notes of the shifts and changes you notice in yourself. Positive changes can easily slip from your awareness before you have the time to reinforce them, so noticing and appreciating them is an important way to touch up your motivation as you progress.

Dig In: What Specific Behaviors Do I Want to Change?

Take a few moments to focus on what it is about your body or behaviors that you specifically want to change. What are you doing that you wish you weren't? Writing down your thoughts will help you gain clarity. Be as specific as possible.

For example, when thinking about what habits you specifically want to change, you may come up with realizations such as "I obsessively count calories and exercise to exhaustion." "I eat uncontrollably." "I eat until I am uncomfortable or immobile." "I eat when I am tired." "I eat to reward myself." "Feelings of guilt and shame accompany every meal I eat—I say horrible things to myself that I'd never say to anyone else." "I starve myself all day and overeat at night." "I eat too fast." "I hide and sneak food." "I binge on sweets and high-fat foods." "I do not shop for groceries or prepare meals." "I waste money on expensive junk food." "I eat when I'm not hungry." "I feel compelled to clean my plate and not waste food." "I feel out of control around food." "I think about food and my weight constantly." Dig in and identify what behaviors and habits you currently have around food and would like to change.

I know, I said that weight release must be enjoyable if it's going to last, and this first exercise is probably anything but that. All the honest introspection, already! I understand that it's no fun to document your current state when you're not happy with it, but it's an important step for creating immediate and lasting motivation. So as tempting as it may be to try to wriggle out of doing it, just start writing. Plus, the chances are high that over the years you've already dedicated a lot of brainpower to what you want to change about yourself. I'm simply asking you to name your undesirable habits out loud and take ownership of them. As uncomfortable or unnecessary as this exercise may seem, it will do you a lot of good in the days and weeks ahead.

Someone Who Tried This Before You

Rosemary came to work with me after years of struggling with her weight on her own. As a housewife whose youngest had recently left home, she felt it was now time to focus on her weight struggle, which had always seemed to be an immovable obstacle in her life. When I asked her what triggered her to overeat, she replied that any situation whatsoever could cause her to overdo it. She was stumped. She felt that there was no pattern at all to her overeating, except that she had no willpower. I asked her to tell me about the last time she had overeaten. She said, "That's easy. Earlier today at the lunch buffet at my club, I ate way past full. They have the most amazing desserts, especially their apple pie."

I said, "Okay, that's good awareness. So you overdid it on the apple pie?"

"Yes," she replied, "and I could have eaten more."

"How much apple pie could you have eaten?" I asked.

"I think I could have eaten about seven of them," she said.

"Slices?" I asked.

"No, pies!" she said. "I just love apple pie, and I can't resist it!"

I was truly impressed by her dedication and commitment to apple pie, and then, to help her become a little more clear on the specific behavior she would like to change, I requested that she slow down her experience from earlier that day at the buffet and asked her what she would have liked to have done instead. She admitted that she would have liked to have eaten just the entrée and skipped dessert. Yet she seemed very sad as she told me that, almost as if giving up dessert altogether would be like losing a dear friend.

Knowing that she would unlikely be able to make a behavior change that felt as depressing as someone's death, we identified two behaviors she'd be willing to change. One was her compulsion to overdo it at a buffet table; the other was her compulsion to consume large quantities of dessert, especially apple pie! *Specific desired behaviors to change: eating past full at the buffet table and overdoing it on desserts.*

How Big Is the Impact?

In addition to identifying the eating habits you want to change, spend another few minutes thinking about how those very behaviors may be affecting your life in other ways. For example, if you're prone to periods of bingeing followed by starving, you may have several wardrobes to accommodate your up-and-down weight. If you feel out of control around food, perhaps you avoid social situations where you think you might overeat. Again, you see where I'm going here? I want you to identify the specific impact of your unhealthful eating habits. For example, does your poor body image carry over into your work performance? Your love life? Have you really put yourself out there in life the way you would have if you truly felt good about yourself and your body? Maybe the impact is even more acute, such as discovering that you're prediabetic or your knees are giving out on you.

I once had a client who wore dark jeans and an oversize T-shirt to work every day. She referred to it as her "uniform" and chose it even though it looked dumpy, because it camouflaged her body. She said it made her look unobjectionable. I questioned her about this, and we discovered that at a deeper and more honest level, she objected to how she was presenting herself to the world. Even though she wanted more, she was afraid and somehow convinced that she didn't deserve to be noticed. She eventually realized that her poor body image not only had taken over her wardrobe but had also hijacked her confidence and was hurting her career.

Are you, too, trying to disappear into the background of your own life? Think about the ways your weight struggle is manifesting itself in all areas of your life and dig into the exercise below. Record your insights in your Full-Filled Weight-Release Journal.

Dig In: What Are My Symptoms?

Take a moment to catalog how the hours when you are not eating are affected by your weight struggle. Identify symptoms—clear outward expressions of your weight struggle—and write them down in your weight-release journal. For example, "I'm forty pounds overweight." "I'm uncomfortable in my body." "I wear unflattering clothes to cover myself up." "I have multiple wardrobes to accompany my up-and-down weight." "I feel self-conscious." "I stay home when I could go out." "I eat alone instead of with people." "I avoid sex." "I lack self-confidence at work." "I have difficulty walking up stairs." "My cholesterol is high." "I am tired and depressed." "I don't want to work out." "I feel old." "Because of my weight struggle, I am putting my life on hold."

Big-Time Consequences

Next, take a look at the consequences of your behaviors. Particularly, how are the people in your life affected by your weight struggle? Romantically, is your relationship suffering because you avoid intimacy? If you're embarrassed by your size, maybe you stay away from romantic relationships altogether and find yourself single when you'd rather not be. Do you compromise your friendships by cancelling social plans because you're afraid of how much you might eat in public or how you look? On the professional front, have you advanced in your career the way you would like to? Perhaps you've been passed over for a promotion because you don't do the job you're capable of, or maybe you haven't even pursued the career of your dreams because you are so afraid of rejection and failure.

Finally, what's going on at home? If you have kids, they will model what you do, even if you do it in secret. I once had a client who became bulimic in her midforties. She kept her bulimia a secret, confiding only in me. Not long after we began working together, her brother was suddenly hospitalized for—bulimia. She'd had no idea he shared a similar secret. She then discovered that both her mother and her aunt had been bulimic, too, and even though she hadn't known consciously of their hidden binges, she and her brother had copied them in adulthood! People often ask me how to help kids lose weight. The best advice is: model the behavior you want them to adopt. Kids will do what you do, so healing and changing yourself will make the biggest difference to their health and well-being.

Dig In: Who's Affected by Your Weight Struggle?

Take a moment to catalog how the people in your life are affected by your weight struggle. Write down your insights. For example, "I am not in a satisfying relationship." "My marriage suffers because I avoid sex." "I'm teaching my kids unhealthy eating habits." "My kids are embarrassed by my size." "I let my boss and my coworkers down by my lack of productivity." "My high/low blood sugar affects my ability to think clearly and solve problems at work." "I'm preoccupied with my weight and not present with other people." "I shy away from meeting new people." "I'm not making good memories with the people I do let into my life." "I'm pushing people away because I'm unhappy and grumpy."

Once you've completed the three lists that catalog the behaviors, symptoms, and consequences of your weight struggle, take a look at what you've written down and spend some additional thought on where this path is taking you. Do you have a clear picture of the future you're creating? As Stephen Covey's *The 7 Habits of Highly Effective People* says, "Your habits define you. Time passes quickly in the status quo. Bring your future in close and look at what you are creating now." If you continue as you are now, what will your future look like? Take a peek at one year from now. How do you feel about yourself? What opportunities have you missed? What's the state of your relationships? How is your health? Zoom out five years down the road. Assuming nothing has changed, what does your life look like? How do you feel? How's your self-esteem? Now imagine maintaining the status quo for another ten years. Do you like what you see?

I'm guessing your answer is no.

The frightening reality is that your future will look nearly identical to your present-day life, only magnified by one, five, ten, or twenty years, unless you change course *now,* so consider this your official wake-up call. If you needed any more convincing that you want to create a better life for yourself, the Dig In exercises you just completed should do the trick. Now, before you slip into paralyzing despair or beat yourself up for all the "wasted years," as one client referred to the time she'd spent struggling with her weight, understand that from this moment forward, you will begin the deep, healing work that will put you on a new course towards a healthy, fulfilling future. So take a deep breath. You're going to be okay. In fact, you're going to be a whole lot better than okay!

Food for Thought

My father used to say to me, "Renée, just remember that it always appears darkest . . . just before it gets pitch black!" He always did have a sense of humor. You may be feeling pretty down right now, after taking a sobering look at the reality of your life today and the future you're creating. Still, take responsibility for it, and then turn it inside out so that it becomes powerful motivation to make positive changes that will transform you into the person you want to be. Let this wake-up call become the fire that fuels you to participate in this process, that gets you going, and that hardens your resolve to make change happen now!

What's Your Motivation?

To get you started down the path that will carry you towards a slim and healthy future, you need powerful motivation. Understandably, you may have had loads of motivation to be slim and healthy in the past, but let me ask you this: how far did it get you? If your motivation started out strong and then pooped out, it's likely that you didn't have the right mix of motivation. You see, not all motivation is created equal. To enjoy permanent, reliable physical change, you need what I call a motivation cocktail, one that is equal parts "away-from" motivation and "towards" motivation.

Understanding Away-from Motivation

Away-from motivation is what motivates people to make declarative statements such as "Starting tomorrow, I'm going on a diet, joining the gym, and never eating like that again!" Away-from motivation is likely what motivated you to pick up this book. It's the motivation to change right here, right now.

Grab your Full-Filled Weight-Release Journal. Look back over your lists of unwanted behaviors, symptoms, and consequences from the section above. Not fun, is it? Gaining that kind of clarity and insight can be very uncomfortable. Realizing that you're pushing away people in your life because of your weight struggle or that you've created a wardrobe to hide your body is painful, and pain is at the heart of away-from motivation. It's the kind of motivation that makes you want to move far and fast away from whatever is causing you to feel emotionally or physically lousy. The lists that you just completed form the basis of your away-from motivation because they have individually and collectively created a reality that I'm guessing you want to move fast and far away from.

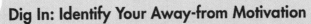

Dig In: Identify Your Away-from Motivation

Refer back to your lists of the unwanted behaviors, symptoms, and consequences of your weight struggle. Based on your lists, write a very clear away-from motivation, starting with "I want to move away from . . ." For example, "I want to move away from overeating when I'm home alone at night." "I want to move away from feelings of guilt and self-loathing." "I want to move away from feeling like my clothes never fit right." "I want to move away from avoiding social interactions because of my fear I'll overeat."

Identifying your away-from motivation is a surefire way to get you revved up for serious change, but it will get you only so far, and that's because motivation that is based solely on pain wears off because the pain wears off before you've reached your ultimate goal. Sound familiar? I bet it does, because we've all been there. Recall an instance where you overate, felt terrible, and swore, "Never again!" Your determination to make drastic change is always rock solid right after you blow it or when you discover you can't button your pants anymore.

In situations such as those, you want to get far and fast away from feeling like a "big fat pig," so you desperately seek a quick fix, a way to lose weight as fast as possible so the pain will go away. That's the appeal of drastic diet plans. *Lose 20 pounds in a month!* We want results, and we want them fast, not in three months, six months, or a year—but by tomorrow morning. Maybe you want to lose 10, 20, or 50 pounds to really feel comfortable in your skin again, but it will take only 5 pounds to get you back into your pants and fasten the button. If your motivation is only an away-from motivation, you'll likely take off just enough weight to fit back into your favorite jeans, and then you'll slack off because the immediate threat is gone. You decide it's okay to have "just one bite" of a cookie or "just a chip or two," and before you know it, you're headfirst into the food and back up on the scale.

Away-from motivation is powerful, but the problem with relying only on that kind of motivation is that once the pain fades (whether in an hour, a day, a week, or a month), the probability of returning to your old habits and regaining the weight you've lost, if you've managed to lose any, is extraordinarily high—if not a certainty. Plus, drastic diet plans powered by away-from motivation are pretty darn miserable. Why? Because in addition to the extreme restrictions of the plan itself, emotionally you have to stay focused on the pain—that is, how bad you feel about yourself—to stay motivated. Most of us can power through like this for a while, but eventually, distraught by what seem to be relentless deprivation, discipline, and abuse, we give up because we're tired of feeling bad. We want to feel good again, and what's a quick, surefire way to feel good? Eating!

Let me give you an extreme example of how away-from motivation can have a boomerang effect. Bulimics, people who binge on huge quantities of food and then purge, are strongly away-from motivated. After a binge, bulimics are so disgusted with themselves for overeating (strong away-from motivation) that they feel an urgent need to escape the pain of self-loathing, plus soothe the physical pain of being so stuffed. They purge as a way to get away from all that horrible pain. But then, as soon as they do this, they feel disgusted with themselves for purging and look for a way to escape that pain (strong away-from motivation again) and feel better. So they turn back to the food. Eating soothes and provides a temporary escape from negative feelings, but it's just a Band-Aid, and as soon as the positive feelings fade, they're back in the bathroom purging. It's a painful cycle.

Away-from motivation is very powerful to get you moving, but it can't take you all the way to your dream body and your dream life. To get to the proverbial promised land, you need another type of motivation.

Understanding Towards Motivation

The most effective, lasting motivation is a combination of "away-from" and "towards" motivation. Towards motivation picks up where your away-from motivation drops off, and it's fueled entirely by what you want. So ask yourself, "Now that I know what I want to move away from, what is it that I want to move towards? What's my dream?" Your towards motivation will move you towards it. Identifying your towards motivation is like creating the master plan for your new slim and healthy life. Having a plan is important. If you hired an architect to design and build your dream home and your only direction was to "create anything except for what I have now, because I really hate it," he'd have no idea where to start. If you want to build a new house for yourself—meaning if you want to create a new body and a new life—you have to be clear about what you want. I wonder, do you know what that is? Do you even know what's possible?

great deal of neck pain due to arthritis. Her pain was so great that it was interfering with her ability to exercise and move in general. Her away-from motivation was that she simply wanted the pain to stop—she wanted to move far and fast away from her discomfort. Fair enough. Yet I challenged her to identify what she wanted instead of the pain. I said, "If you could replace the pain with something else, what would it be?" After some thought, she realized that what she truly wanted was a feeling of flexibility and openness in her neck. This became her towards motivation, and after she'd identified it, we spent the remainder of our session focused solely on the feeling of flexibility and openness she desired.

Guess what happened next? The weekend following our session, she went to yoga class—an activity she did regularly and enjoyed even though it had never before alleviated her chronic neck pain. That time, however, she went in with focused intent and towards motivation to experience openness and flexibility in her neck. She left the class that day feeling pain-free for the first time in years! Moreover, she became more flexible in the days and weeks afterward because she'd identified a clear intention in her mind for her body to follow.

Knowing what you want not only is liberating, it actually starts to take you there. So what is it that you want? Have you ever thought about that? How you answer this question is very important in determining what you will get. If I say to you, "Don't think about a flabby cottage-cheese butt," what do you think of? A flabby cottage-cheese butt! It's irresistible. The subconscious mind, which runs the show when it comes to automatic behavior, doesn't understand negative commands. It ignores words such as "don't" and "not" and just hears the dominant action command and immediately starts to enact it. So if you say to yourself, "Don't be bad. Don't eat. Don't even think about food," what does your subconscious mind hear? "Eat. Eat. Eat!" Saying "I don't want to eat sweets" to yourself is like giving yourself an order to eat sweets all day long. Talk about counterproductive!

A friend of mine said she was fighting off a bug that was going around her office. She told me she'd been repeating to herself, "Don't get sick, don't get sick" for several days but felt it was inevitable that she'd come down with the collective cold. After I pointed out that she'd actually been telling herself to get sick, she changed her tune and began repeating, "Be healthy, be healthy," and she beat the cold bug. So when thinking about your towards motivation, be mindful of stating your answer in the positive. In other words, say what you want, instead of what you don't want. For instance, say, "I *want to move towards* slimness. I *am moving towards* slimness." You will be amazed and delighted by the impact this simple change will make on your life.

Dig In: What Is Your Towards Motivation?

What is the life you want to create? Write your answer in the positive. In other words, say what you want, starting with "I want to move towards . . ." For example, "I want to move towards being so healthy that I'm med-free" or "I want to move towards wearing my stylish clothes again" or "I want to move towards eating moderately." Resist the temptation to state what you don't want, such as "I don't want to have to take medication," "I don't want to have to buy a bigger, frumpy wardrobe," or "I don't want to eat junk food late at night." Identify the motivation that will pull you forward on your weight loss journey.

If identifying your towards motivation seems difficult, relax. It takes practice. Even I'm still challenged from time to time, and I've been working with this system for more than ten years. Most of us dieters are so conditioned to focus on what we *don't* want that thinking about what we *do* want can throw us for a loop. You think, "What I really want is to not eat, so how do I state that in the positive?" Typically, the first few times my clients try this exercise, they create a long list of "don't wants" disguised as "do wants" without realizing it. Take this statement, for example: "I want to eat dinner without overstuffing myself." This is actually a negative command. To restate this in the positive, you might say, "I want to eat dinner until my body feels just satisfied."

Food for Thought

Most of us are so conditioned to think of the negative, of what we don't want and don't like, that it can take some real effort to figure out what we want instead. After all, the vast majority of news reporting focuses on negativity: crime, bad economic news, wars, terrorism, and a seemingly endless array of things to be outraged about. So if you find yourself stumped when you ask, "What do I want?" simply start with what you don't want and ask yourself what the opposite of that is. Then fine-tune to create the dream that's just right for you.

The trick is to turn the statement around so that it includes the presence of something else. Practice restating negatives into positives by making a two-column list in your Full-Filled Weight-Release Journal. On one side, list your "don't wants" ("I don't want to undress in front of people at the gym because I'm embarrassed about how I look"); on the other side, transform your statement into a "do want" ("I want to move towards feeling comfortable getting undressed in front of people at the gym"). See the difference?

I don't want . . .	Instead I want to move towards . . .
_____	_____
_____	_____
_____	_____
_____	_____
_____	_____

Note: As a bonus, reframing your statements in the positive is a great parenting strategy. If you tell your kids what not to do, the surest thing they'll do is exactly what you said not to. That isn't because your children are little hellions who have it out for you, but because they are predominantly ruled by their subconscious minds. They hear your command—"Don't eat in the living room"—but ignore the "don't" because that's how the subconscious mind works. To restate this command in the positive, you might say, "Please eat all your meals and snacks at the kitchen table."

Someone Who Tried This Before You

Liane is a client who started her weight-release journey with a strong away-from motivation. At sixty-three, she was morbidly obese and unable to walk without experiencing severe pain. Her away-from motivation was to move away from being disabled by her size. This away-from motivation was strong enough to motivate her to drop 30 pounds and undergo knee replacement surgery. Once she was back on her feet, Liane's away-from motivation faded in intensity, so she needed a towards motivation to keep her going. She became excited about walking the block and a half uphill from her house to the park. Reaching that goal became her new motivation—and it pulled her forward one step at a time. It took her several months, but once she was able to make the walk to the top of the hill and back with ease, she set a new intention for herself. Over time, she tackled every hill in her neighborhood. She released an additional 100 pounds, and eventually, being mobile and active, as well as feeling good in her body each day, became her ongoing towards motivation. Liane eventually dropped to and stabilized at 135 pounds, a slim and healthy weight that she's maintained for four years!

♥

Tanya arrived at my office flustered and exhausted. She was just nine months into a demanding new job and had already gained 20-plus pounds since starting. She confided that she had only one or two pieces of clothing left in her closet that still fit. She was disgusted by her recent weight gain yet felt unable to get her stress eating under control. Her mornings at work were consumed by an obsession with lunch, and her afternoons were spent feeling guilty for overeating at midday.

As we began speaking about what motivated her, she was quick to say that she wanted to move fast and far away from obsessing about food, gaining weight uncontrollably, and growing out of her wardrobe. In addition, she felt she was becoming reclusive and antisocial because she was too embarrassed by her weight to be seen out. She really wanted to change her social behavior as well.

I then asked her what she wanted instead of the obsession with food, the reclusiveness, and the suffering. She began to evaluate her decisions and noticed a gap between the way she was behaving and who she really was. She concluded that she wanted to be her "self" again—a vibrant, energetic person who enjoyed life and was surrounded by friends and loved ones. That desire became her towards motivation.

To help her move towards her intention, I suggested she begin making social time and downtime a top priority. She stopped working late into the night and over the weekends. With more hours in the day to work on herself, she found time to get back into an exercise routine and reconnect with friends. After she shifted away from all work and no play and towards a more balanced schedule, her overeating became less frequent and intense. The pounds began to come off, and a vibrant, energetic, and full life became her ongoing towards motivation.

Create Your Dream Future

Your towards motivation will be what pulls you forward over the next six weeks and towards your dream life, so take your time thinking about what you truly want. And while you're doing so, allow yourself to dream big. Have some fun. I really want you to let yourself go here. Albert Einstein said, "Your imagination is your preview of life's coming attractions." Give yourself permission to dream about the future you want; it should be one that excites you, that you're passionate about, and that makes you think, "*Yes!*"

For example, a vivacious client in her sixties wanted to turn heads on the street. "I want to be noticed for how amazing I look," she said. Another client had always dreamed of traveling but had reluctantly stayed put because she didn't want to be ostracized for her size. Her towards motivation was to fit into a single airline seat so she could travel the world. After working the Full-Filled program, she spent six months in Europe and Africa. Another client was ashamed and embarrassed about how her body looked in a swimsuit. Her towards motivation was to feel confident in a one-piece so she could play with her daughter on the beach without fretting over how she looked to those around her. And that's exactly what she achieved—and much sooner than she expected.

Food for Thought

What if your dreams are too big? I've had clients tell me they are actually afraid of how powerful or attractive they would be if they slimmed down. Maybe you, too, already get a lot of attention and have no idea how you would handle it if you got more. Or perhaps you're afraid of how your friends or family would react to you if you lost your excess weight. For now, let all of this go and give yourself permission to dream big—we'll address any fears you might have next week. Or, if your dreams really are overwhelming, choose an interim dream for now. You can always dream bigger later on. Just make sure your dream is something that excites you and pulls you towards it.

When you're creating your towards motivation, you'll want to mix up long-term motivation, like Liane's block-and-a-half uphill walk, with short-term motivators, such as simply eating three moderate meals a day and feeling good in your body after every one. I'm sure you agree that feeling so full that it hurts is a lousy way to spend your time, and beating yourself up because your clothes don't fit the way you want them to can ruin a perfectly good morning. So in addition to identifying your long-term towards motivation, think about day-to-day, short-term motivators that will pull you forward, too, like the endorphin rush after a really great workout or the enjoyable feeling of putting your fork down when you're just satisfied. One of my personal favorite short-term motivators is waking up with a good appetite because it means I ate a healthful amount of food the night before, and I'll really enjoy my breakfast. Have you ever noticed that food tastes so much better when we eat when we're hungry? Plus, when I eat only until I'm satisfied—not stuffed—I get to feel really good in my body for hours afterward. Find daily short-term motivators that give you pleasure, make you feel good, and also pull you towards your long-term intention.

Someone Who Tried This Before You

Sue was a successful pediatrician and married with two children. Born in Korea, she had always been driven to achieve by her mother, and as a result, now that she lived in the United States, she was always working towards the next higher qualification. Her days were filled with taking care of her patients and her family, as well as studying for the next big exam. On top of that, she managed to call her mother, who still lived in Korea, every day to check in. And like clockwork, as soon as she hung up with her mother, she'd head face-first into the snacks. Every day, she found herself eating to dull the ache of yet another unsatisfying conversation with her mother.

Sue's long-term motivation was to drop 30 to 40 pounds, yet the goal seemed far off to her and extremely difficult to attain. As we talked about her towards motivation and her long-term intentions, she realized that her conversations with her mother almost always triggered her to overeat (as did her yearly trips to Korea, which she would invariably spend eating and gaining weight). She never felt as though she met her mother's high expectations and was constantly working to prove herself but was never successful.

I asked her, "What's one situation that you could change that would make the biggest positive difference for you?" She quickly realized that if she could stop eating after her daily chats with her mom, she would consume a lot less calories in a day. So she set a short-term intention of passing on the snacks after her daily call with her mother and finding simple activities, such as taking a walk outside or sinking into a hot bath, to feel good about herself immediately afterward instead. This new short-term motivator helped her consume less on a daily basis and also empowered her to begin separating her own self-worth from her mother's preconceived judgments of her.

Put Your Inner Critic on Hold

If imagining your dream future feels like a waste of your time because it will never happen, know that you're having a very normal response. Most of us dieters have trained ourselves to ratchet down our dreams because we've had so much disappointment in the past. Because we've struggled for so long comparing ourselves to others and battling with self-hatred when we don't succeed in the ways we'd hoped, dreaming of success feels like a ticket to disappointment. It becomes easier and safer to not dream at all. Yet the deeper, longer-lasting burn is that, when we don't dream, our dreams can't come true. Now, that's no way to dream, is it?

In Week 3, you'll learn how important and necessary your "screw-ups" are to becoming slim and healthy for a lifetime. But at this stage of the game, it's important simply to let your dreamer dream without input from your inner critic. You know the voice I'm talking about, right? It's the one that tells you that dreaming is a waste of your time because you're destined to be overweight and unhappy. It's the voice that whispers, "I'll never be able to change. I'll never fit in. I'll always look the way I do because I'm just a big-boned person. My mother was fat, my father was fat, my cousin is fat, and my dog is fat, so I am always going to be fat."

Food for Thought

Walt Disney, the man who invented the modern theme park and introduced countless animated classics to the screen, was an expert at turning dreams into reality. He used to say that though he didn't know exactly what the future held, he knew that it was bright and beautiful and shimmering as it drew him towards it. If you don't yet have the specifics of your dream self, enjoy what you do have, perhaps a feeling or a bright, shimmering image, and allow the rest, especially the steps for how to get there, to come into focus as you go. Often we demand that our dreams come with complete operating instructions, including how to get from here to there. We'll get to the how soon enough. For now it's time just to dream.

As hard as it may be, you must, must, *must* put the critic that says your dreams are unrealistic or unattainable on hold while you give yourself permission to dream. By keeping your critical voice thoroughly separated from your inner dreamer, you will tap into the courage that allows you to go for what you truly and deeply desire. If, while you're dreaming, your critic speaks up, simply say to it, "Thank you very much, I'm just going to turn the volume down on your voice and ask you to wait on hold while I dream my dream and plan my plan." Next week, you will ask your inner critic what objections it has to your dream, but for now—simply turn down the voice and dream big.

Below is a short meditation to help you fully experience what it is that you want so much. Take a moment to relax and drop inside before doing the following mindful meditation, "Step into Your Future Self."

 ### Mindful Meditation: Step into Your Future Self

Begin by imagining what it is that you truly want. Is it fitting back into all the clothes in your closet and turning heads on the street? Maybe you dream of your body regulating its blood sugar perfectly, having endless energy and resilient health, and throwing away your meds because you don't need them anymore. Perhaps your dream is to get to a place where you feel perfectly at ease around food and where you eat only when you're hungry and automatically stop when you're full.

Whatever it is, begin to think about that now; in fact, what I'd like you to do is imagine trying on your ideal self. Notice the details. How is it that you look? Imagine looking into a mirror and seeing your reflection. Imagine someone else noticing how you look. You're slim, you're attractive, you're healthy. No more muffin top. No more huffing and puffing. Only health, wellness, and well-being. As you think about that, I want you to imagine the you who already has what you want standing right there in front of you. Make sure your vision of yourself is of a future you, not the you of five, ten, or fifteen years ago, when you last were the weight you want to be today. This program is about moving forward. The future you is new and improved—wiser, more mature. You have what you want, and it's better and more stable than ever before.

Do you have an image of the future you in your mind? In a moment you're going to step in and become that person. Doing this while standing is especially powerful, so stand up right now. If you're not in a place where you can stand up, vividly imagine doing it in your head.

Ready?

1 . . .

2 . . .

3 . . .

→ Step in.

Wow! This is it. This is what you've been dreaming of. Now that you've become the person you want to be, notice what it feels like. You've got it now. Do you feel more energetic? More alive? Do you feel as though a burden has been lifted from you? Now notice the sound of your inner voice. Is it still making critical comments, or has it softened? Perhaps it's taken on the tone of a good friend. Imagine how you behave now that you're the new you. Are you more active? What foods do you choose to eat? Do you grocery shop regularly? Go to your local farmers' market? Do you have good friends whom you share a fitness routine with? Do you take time out for you? Finally, what kind of thoughts do you have? What goes on in your head? Do you believe you're worthy of patience, praise, and care? Do you believe that being slim and healthy is easy and enjoyable and that you can keep the weight off without a struggle? Every behavior begins with a thought. By imagining your future self with your senses—seeing, hearing, and feeling—you make it more real and actually start creating it!

As you come to the end of Week 1 of the Full-Filled program, spend a few moments thinking about your two possible futures: the one you've been creating through your current habits and behaviors, and the future you truly want. I'd like you to think about your dream future and notice very carefully—do you like it? Really, do you like what you see? This might seem like a funny question to ask, but the reality is, if all of you wanted it, you'd already have it by now.

So what's stopping you?

Progress Report

This program is all about working at your own pace, but as you make your way through each week of the Full-Filled program, you will be provided with a weekly Progress Report to help you stay on track and motivated towards reliable and lasting change. Once you've checked each item off your list, you'll know that you're making significant progress and you're good and ready to move on to the next week of the Full-Filled program.

Over the next seven days, be sure to:

1. **Begin a Full-Filled Weight-Release Journal** that you will keep by your side for the next six weeks. A written progress report will help keep you accountable for your actions and help you track your thoughts and eating habits as they change. In Week 1, there were five Dig In exercises. Did you complete them all? Did you write your insights down? If not, go back through them and make notes on each exercise before moving on to Week 2 of the program. Imagine how great it will be at the end of six weeks to look back and see all the progress you have made.

2. **Take a mental and an actual snapshot of yourself.** Paste this photo into your weight-release journal. I know, it's not fun. But just think about how great it will feel to look back at the photo in the near future and see how far you've come. Give this gift to yourself.

3. **Join or create your own support group.** Your group could be as small as a party of two—you and your BFF—or a larger group of ten or more. It could be online or offline. It doesn't really matter as long as you surround yourself with a community. Research

proves it: when you enlist outside support, you create a system of encouragement and accountability that dramatically accelerates your progress and keeps you on track towards reliable and permanent change.

4. **Determine where you are now and why you want to change.** Catalog in your weight-release journal the specific eating behaviors unique to you that you want to change. How are those behaviors affecting other areas of your life? Is your health compromised? Is your self-esteem suffering? And what people in your life—colleagues, family, friends, lovers—are being affected by your weight struggle?

5. **Recognize and create your away-from motivation.** This is the kind of motivation that makes you want to move far and fast away from whatever is causing you to feel emotionally or physically lousy. Identify your away-from motivation and write it down in your weight-release journal. For example, "I want to move away from having a food hangover in the mornings." "I want to move away from feelings of guilt and self-loathing." "I want to move away from turning down social invitations because I feel too fat." List in your weight-release journal what isn't working and what you want less of in your life.

6. **Recognize and create your towards motivation.** Your towards motivation picks up where your away-from motivation drops off, and it's fueled entirely by what you want. What is the life you want to create? Write your answer in the positive. Say what you want instead of what you don't want. For example, "I want to move towards being so fit and healthy that I can run a 10k." When creating your towards motivation, be sure to mix long-term motivation with short-term motivators, such as simply feeling good in your body each day.

7. **Vividly imagine your dream future and your dream self.** How do you look? Feel? What kinds of thoughts go through your head on a daily basis? How has your lifestyle changed? Remember to put your inner critic on hold while you dream your dream. The

important thing about turning your future dream into reality is to keep your critical voice separated from your dreamer. Over the next seven days, spend some time vividly imagining your dream self in different scenarios and notice if any objections come up. Write down those insights.

Put a Stop to Your Internal Tug-of-War

Do you know what's stopping you from creating the life and body of your dreams? Do you know what's getting in your way? The truth is, if all of you really wanted to be slim and healthy, you would be. Forgive me if that sounds harsh, but it's true. If you really wanted the dream you just finished imagining for yourself, you wouldn't be sneaking and snacking on high-fat foods and stuffing yourself until your pants don't button.

So tell me, what's your objection to becoming slim and healthy for a lifetime? Do you know what it is?

Maybe you didn't realize you have an objection and my suggestion that you do has you yelling in protest into this very page— "Renée, I do want to be slim and healthy! Don't you think I would be if I could be?"

Yes and no.

That you don't already have the body and life you want tells me that some part of you objects to actually getting it. Though part of you is all for being slim and healthy, there's another part of you that says, "One more cookie won't hurt." In short, you're in conflict— big-time inner conflict. And until you resolve your internal tug-of-war, you won't be able to create the life and body of your dreams. Relax. You will resolve this conflict by *evolving* through it.

In Week 2 of the Full-Filled program, you will:

- Identify your objection to becoming slim and healthy for a lifetime
- Discover what you're getting out of your current eating habits
- Learn why the cycle of overeating is often so hard to break
- Resolve your internal tug-of-war

What's Your Objection?

As you begin Week 2 of the Full-Filled program, **set the intention to identify the objection or objections that are holding you back from becoming the person of your dreams.** Take a deep, cleansing breath, and set this intention right now. For example, "My intention is to identify any and all objections that are holding me back and keeping me from becoming my dream self."

Many of my first-time clients tell me, "I don't understand it. I'm successful in so many other areas of my life. It's just with eating that I can't seem to control myself. I've tried everything, and nothing seems to work. Why can't I lose weight and keep it off?" What's often standing in their way is their unconscious objections to releasing weight. Once we begin to explore their personal objections to weight loss, they get it.

Over the years, clients have shared all sorts of objections with me. And you know what? I've never met an objection I didn't like. I've heard them all, including:

"If I finally lose the last fifteen pounds, I'll have to face what else is wrong with me."

"I'm afraid of succeeding and then failing all over again. If I just maintain the status quo, I won't have to deal with the disappointment of losing my extra weight only to regain it all back."

"I'm comfortable being not 'good enough.' If people don't have high expectations of me, I don't have to work very hard."

"I get a lot of attention for my 'woe is me' attitude. I have a lot of friends with food/weight issues, and we spend a lot of our time talking about these issues. If I no longer struggle with my weight, I worry that we'll have less to talk about. I might even lose my friends."

"My mother has always suffered with her weight. I need to suffer, too, so we can have that bond and connection. Somehow I'd be betraying her if I was happy and she wasn't."

"If I become slimmer and more attractive, I'll be more noticeable. I go back and forth between wanting to be visible and wanting to hide from the world."

"I just don't feel safe. The truth is that I get a lot more attention from men when I'm slim, and I don't like it. Being overweight is safe for me."

"I don't trust myself. When I was thinner and more attractive in the past, I wasn't faithful in my relationships. I don't want to blow it with the great guy I have now."

"My weight gives me more 'weight' to throw around. If I were slimmer, maybe people wouldn't take me as seriously in the workplace."

"Part of living a slim and healthful lifestyle means going to the gym, and I can't stand looking at myself in all those full-length mirrors. It's horrifying!"

"I'm afraid that I won't be able to handle life's pressures and stress without food."

"Food is like a good friend. She comforts me in times of need. How will I cope when I don't have my trusted friend to entertain, comfort, and reassure me, and to distract me from uncomfortable situations?"

"My dream feels unknown and scary. If I become slimmer, I'm afraid I won't know who I am anymore."

"My dream feels too big. It's a lot of pressure."

"What if I don't lose enough weight? Or what if I lose all my excess weight only to regain it? Then people will judge me more than they already do now."

"If I lose weight, people will start commenting on 'how good I look,' and I'll have to acknowledge how fat I was before. How depressing!"

As you can see, there are all sorts of objections you might have to becoming your dream self. While the act of dreaming feels safe, to imagine really becoming that person can scare the bejeebers out of us. It turns out that our dreams often come with objectionable consequences. When I was still struggling with food, though I very much wanted to break free, a part of me was terrified. If I were finally slim, I'd have no excuse left for why I wasn't living up to my full potential. And if I didn't measure up, I'd be seen as a failure. It was my stubborn perfectionism that objected to losing weight. As long as I was still struggling, the pressure was off me to be perfect. On one side of my internal tug-of-war was the desire to be slim and healthy; on the other was fear of screwing up and being seen as the flawed, imperfect person I am.

I had a client who was more than 100 pounds overweight. Though she very much wanted to be slimmer, she objected to releasing her excess weight because it would mean that she'd have to face the fact that she had "let herself go." On one side of her internal tug-of-war was the desperate desire to be slim and healthy so she could be more present for her kids and her life; on the other was resistance to accept what she'd become. She had great shame, regret, and sadness about her weight gain, and by remaining inactive and resistant to change, she created a coping mechanism for her pain.

Now it's your turn. Identify any objection that's holding you back. Find a private, quiet place where you can relax and reflect without interruption and dig into the exercise below. Write down your answers in the journal you've dedicated to your weight-release journey. Also, after you've completed all the Dig In exercises for this second week of the Full-Filled program, set aside some time to check in with your support community online or offline and share your new insights. If you haven't joined or created a support community yet, make it a priority this week. My Inside Out Weight Loss Yahoo!

group via my website at www.insideoutweightloss.com is a good place to begin making connections with others who are also on the weight-release journey.

Food for Thought

The more you interact with and participate in this program, the more you'll get out of it. You'll get back many times over what you put in, but you *must* put in to get out. Releasing weight from the inside out is not a passive transformation. Make a commitment today to engaging and participating with others, to learning from and supporting others who are on a similar journey.

Dig In: Notice Your Objections

Close your eyes and imagine your ideal self. Go back to the image from Week 1 of who it is you truly want to be. What do you physically look like? Remember to make sure you are imagining yourself in the future, not your svelte eighteen-year-old self at senior prom. This is the body you will evolve into in the future. How do you carry yourself? Are you confident? How do you feel in your new body? Are you full of energy? Are you strong?

Once you have a clear picture in your mind of the person you want to become, ask yourself, "Is there any part of me that objects to realizing this dream?" Take your time. Notice your physical body. Are you experiencing any sensations of discomfort? How do you feel in your torso where your emotions reside? Notice any and all thoughts and feelings that come up. Take your time, and notice any objections. What are they? Write them down.

Not as easy as one-two-three? If this exercise feels difficult, relax and try slowing down your mind. Imagine downshifting your brain from fourth gear to third to second to first. Take a deep breath. Close your eyes, and, as you continue to breathe, give yourself permission to let all thoughts, images, and feelings rise to the surface. As thoughts, images, and feelings begin to take form, write down the first thing that pops into your mind. It may be a single word, such as "family," or a feeling, such as "scared." Perhaps an image or a memory comes to mind. As inconsequential or random as it may seem, whatever comes up, make note of it. One client saw herself onstage in a sexy red dress, singing to a huge crowd. Though the idea of performing on stage filled her with excitement, it also scared the pants, *err,* the dress, off of her, but she eventually resolved her objection to becoming her dream self, realizing that singing onstage would be an option she would create for herself if she so chose. Releasing weight didn't mean she had to take to the stage, only that she could.

Food for Thought

Have you ever received a secret gift? Something that surprised and delighted you? Sometimes such gifts come disguised as objections, challenges, and even disasters. Think for a moment of the biggest challenges you have faced in your life. What gifts did you receive from those challenges? Have they made you stronger? Did you learn valuable lessons from them? Did they advance you in ways you couldn't have imagined before?

Whether or not it makes sense to you right now, trust that the message you've given yourself holds significance, and write it down. The objections that hold us back the most are usually the ones that, when said aloud, sound illogical, even ridiculous. So if you feel tempted to dismiss your objection, know that you're onto something profound.

Once you've finished the Dig In exercise, think for a moment about the part of you that is objecting to your dream. Does it sound silly? Absurd? Why on earth would you let this objection hold you back? Why not just give up the struggle and let Team Slim and Healthy win? Have you figured it out? I'll give you a hint: you're objecting to becoming slim and healthy for a lifetime because you're getting something out of your current weight and eating habits. Something you don't want to give up. Something positive!

Positive Intent

Think about it: what if the part of you who overeats and is overweight actually wants something positive for yourself? You probably haven't thought about it this way before because you're so accustomed to beating yourself up. (And I bet you're a master at it!) But at the root of your unhealthful eating habits is something called "positive intent." Behind every action and every behavior you have, there's positive intent. Said a different way, you eat and weigh what you do because you want to feel good. "Duh," you say. "Food tastes good." But that's not what I'm talking about. I'm not referring to the positive feelings that go along with that first decadent bite of triple-layer chocolate cake. I'm talking about a benefit that goes deep below the surface.

Take, for example, my client who was afraid that if she lost her excess weight, she'd no longer be able to relate to her friends who also struggled with weight issues. What do you suppose her positive intent was for keeping her weight up? Acceptance and connection. Eating and weighing what she did allowed her to stay included in the group. In the case of the woman who felt she needed extra weight to throw around the workplace, what was her positive intent? Respect. Though a part of her desperately desired to lose her excess weight, another part of her craved that important nod from her colleagues.

Finally, in the case of the woman who was afraid that a slimmer version of herself would attract the unwelcome attention of men, what do you suppose was her positive intent for staying heavy? Protection. Extra weight, it turns out, is a very common defense in women who have had sexual trauma. Rape victims and victims of sexual abuse often gain weight to appear less attractive, in an attempt to ward off another traumatic attack.

Do you see how in each of those instances my clients were getting something positive out of overeating and being overweight? Though their excess weight was making them very unhappy, they were still getting something out of it that they weren't willing to give up. Those deeper desires often go unnoticed, but once you begin to dig below the surface and discover that positive intent drives every fistful of french fries you put into your mouth, your weight struggle and motivations for overeating will start to make a lot more sense.

Someone Who Tried This Before You

Pam, a thirty-two-year-old marketing executive with an Ivy League MBA, was accustomed to success. Not only did she have a full-time management job, she also had a profitable web-based side business. Yet she was unable to control her eating. She was a secret binger. The same techniques of planning and control that worked so well for her professionally failed her miserably when it came to eating. In fact, it seemed that the more she tried to control her behavior, the worse it became. She came to see me in desperation. "How do I break the cycle?" she asked.

The cause of Pam's problem was that she actually resented the control that ruled her professional life. Her fondest wish was to be more spontaneous and free. Backed into a corner by her demanding schedule and high standards, she found the only outlet for spontaneity and freedom available: uncontrolled eating. Once she discovered that the positive intent of her eating behavior was to give her a sense of freedom and spontaneity, she began to reorganize her life.

Her first step was to move her workday lunch from her desk to the break room. Soon she was craving an even better break and began eating on a bench by the water outside. With each move, she felt less frantic and more relaxed and renewed. She ate more slowly, enjoying each bite more. She began to plan dinners with friends, focusing on their company more and the food less. Eventually her need to binge fell away, and the pounds went, too. By our final session, not only was she not bingeing, she was also enjoying smaller portions. Plus, she'd cut her hours back and was planning her dream sabbatical to do volunteer work with children in Africa.

There are all sorts of things you might be getting out of your eating habits and excess weight. It's time to notice these things. Take a moment now to dig in and uncover the positive intent. Write your insights in your Full-Filled Weight-Release Journal.

Dig In: What Is the Positive Intent of Your Eating Habits?

Think for a moment about the part of you that gets you to overeat, underexercise, and make unhealthful choices. Then close your eyes and ask yourself, "What's really great about overeating? About being overweight? What am I getting out of it?"

Did you just say, "Nothing"? Not true. There's something that you're getting out of being heavy and overeating. Guaranteed. Even when you make yourself sick eating until you can't get up off

> the couch, your intention, believe it or not, is positive. Before the
> negative feelings of discomfort, guilt, or shame set in, you're get-
> ting, or at least seeking, something positive from the immediate
> experience or the eventual outcome. Dig in. Ask the objecting part
> of you, "What is the positive intent of my eating habits?"

If you can't identify it right away, continue to keep your mind open for the answer. It will come. To help you, I've listed below some general overeater personalities I've identified after helping tens of thousands of people just like you. Can you spot yourself in any of them? You may be predominantly one of them but have a secondary personality as well. As you read through, note in your weight-release journal where you recognize yourself.

The Giver

The Giver excels at putting others' needs before her own. She's the selfless mother, the devoted daughter, the loyal friend, and she will give until she has nothing left. Others admire her extraordinary heart and generosity, but try urging her to spend a little less time on others and give more attention to herself. "No, no, no," she objects. "It's better to give than to receive." Underneath it all, she hates to ask for anything because she fears she's unworthy and not deserving of the love and care she bestows on others. For her, giving is a way to be re-deemed. Unfortunately, no matter how much she gives, at the end of the day she still feels unworthy and undeserving. Because self-worth is what she truly desires, she continues to give.

Food helps the Giver in several ways. Her relentless giving leaves her emotionally, spiritually, and physically drained, and eating is an attempt to replenish her energy. As a result, she favors quick-energy-boost foods such as sweets and starches, as well as comfort foods. Her extra weight also serves her because it hides her true, "unworthy" self. The positive intent of her overeating is to recharge so she can keep on giving and to create a physical buffer that hides her true self from the rest of the world.

The Fraud

The Fraud has the overwhelming feeling that, no matter what she does or how hard she tries, underneath it all she's just a fake, a pretender. She's managed to fool everyone up until now, but she feels it's just a matter of time before she's found out. She's always on alert and always fearful, guarding her shameful secret—that she's not good enough, not qualified enough, not up to snuff. Consequently, she is often overprepared and can become extremely defensive when her decisions or behavior is questioned. Always afraid she'll be "found out," she's often conservative in her approach to life, holding herself back from really going for what she wants and experiencing true fulfillment. Safety and security are key for her, and food seems to provide both. Eating works to dampen the pain associated with her feelings of inadequacy, while it momentarily distracts her from facing herself. The positive intents of her overeating are comfort, safety, and security.

The Perfectionist

The Perfectionist holds herself to extremely high standards. Though high standards can be a good thing, in the case of the Perfectionist, they backfire. Because she views anything less than perfection as absolute failure, she's terrified of screwing up. She's always hungry for the approval of others, desperately trying to wow them with her spectacular achievements. The pressure of it all is too much for her, so, as an escape, she procrastinates—better to avoid the task altogether than do it badly. She has an acute fear of failure, disappointment, and judgment, so she eats to distract herself from the pressure of doing her next task perfectly and to put off the inevitable negative judgments that she and others will make. In addition, overeating provides her with a ready scapegoat for not measuring up. "I'd be fabulous if it weren't for my weight," she thinks. The positive intent of her overeating is twofold: it provides relief from the unremitting pressure she puts on herself, and it allows her to procrastinate and, again, put off the inevitable negative judgments about her that others might make. Ultimately, the Perfectionist craves approval.

The Overachieving Multitasker

Like the Perfectionist, the Overachieving Multitasker is what she does. So the more she does, the better person she is. Downtime is for wimps! You'll find her checking her messages on her mobile device while in line at the coffee bar, impatiently tapping her foot. She has multiple projects going at any one time and relentlessly pushes herself to do them all because they are all important. When she decides it's time for a break, she'll come up with a clever way to multitask on her downtime; for instance, she'll work out on the treadmill after dinner while catching up on her business reading. Because downtime is a waste of time in her mind, she eats in a rush, snacks throughout the day, and often overeats to give herself a release from the relentless doing—and get a zap of energy while she's at it. As a result, she often has a weakness for energy boosters such as caffeine, sugar, and refined carbs. Even if she eats at her computer, walking down the street, or in the car on the way to her next meeting, food gives her a small respite from her rigorous schedule because, whether she admits it or not, she's exhausted. Unfortunately, food on the go is no substitute for real rest and quality downtime, but because accomplishment is how she measures self-worth, she always has a new, terribly important task to complete. The positive intent of her overeating is permission to relax and take a break, and to boost her energy so she can keep doing, doing, doing and, ultimately, feel she's successful and worthy of praise.

The Rebel

The Rebel wants to be known as her own person. She resents society for telling her what to eat and not eat and how much she "should" weigh or how she should look. She steadfastly refuses to conform to anyone else's ideal and dislikes authority figures because they are just people who want to control her. Secretly, however, she is afraid she won't be seen for who she really is and is terrified of being ignored, overlooked, or taken advantage of. She wants to do what she wants and still be loved for it, so she tests the world around her. If she "rebels" and overeats, gains weight, and is still accepted, she must really be loved. The positive intent of her overeating is to be recognized, accepted, and loved for who she truly is.

The Abused

The Abused feels safer when she's bigger. She has suffered some kind of abuse or trauma in her past, either emotional or sexual, and as a result she finds the world unsafe. She may be extremely safety conscious, overly worried about security, and conservative sexually. Like the Giver, she uses her weight to create a boundary between herself and the outside world. For the Abused, eating is often an escape from the pain of the trauma, and the extra weight is a way to make herself less attractive to potential attackers, thereby acting as protection. In other cases, the Abused takes on a daredevil persona, taking foolish risks, perhaps becoming sexually promiscuous. Her risky behavior is an attempt to rewrite history and get someone to treat her well. Unfortunately, she will almost always hook up with the same abusive type again. In the end, the positive intent of her weight and overeating is to keep her safe and protected from what she believes is an inherently dangerous world.

The Mystic

The Mystic walks around with her head in the clouds. To others, she seems to live in a different realm. She may be psychic, highly intuitive, or spiritually focused. For her, food and weight are ways to ground her in the here and now. More common perhaps, but often overlooked, is the Reluctant Mystic. She is highly intuitive and doesn't want to be. Supersensitive, she has an excess of empathy and may actually feel other people's emotions. She may also see, hear, or just "know" things. Because she's often overwhelmed by her intuitive nature, the Reluctant Mystic may find crowded spaces, including gyms, restaurants, and social gatherings, especially difficult because of all the energy she's exposed to. Generally, she is overstimulated and often feels responsible for the woes of others, simply because she's hyperaware of them. She worries that she won't be able to handle and process all the information she's picking up on. In reaction to this fear, both the Mystic and the Reluctant Mystic have a tendency to eat uncontrollably and use food to buffer themselves from the barrage of input they are subjected to every day. As they are highly sensitive and susceptible to stress, the positive intent of their overeating is refuge and to ground themselves in the material world.

You may recognize yourself in more than one of these personality types; in fact, several of them overlap. I was the Perfectionist and the Fraud with a hint of the Overachieving Multitasker. Underneath my need to be perfect was a deep fear that I'd be found out for being a fake, a pretender, and ultimately not good or worthy enough. Once you get beneath your own skin and find, identify with, and explore your primary personality type, you may uncover a secondary one as well.

For example, underneath the Giver is often—but not always—the Abused. She uses her giving to try to win the love of others—the love that was painfully absent during her abuse. Similarly, the Rebel and the Abused often overlap. Here the Abused channels her anger over her abuse at anything that represents the establishment. The Overachieving Multitasker often identifies with the Perfectionist *and* the Fraud because her compulsive doing is a way to avoid being "found out" for being less than perfect. The Mystic occasionally overlaps with the Giver; she tries to solve the world's problems with one generous but self-depleting act at a time. At different points in your life and throughout your eating history, you may lean towards different personality types, depending on what you're craving on a deep level.

In addition to noticing some overlap in the general personality types above, can you also recognize that your positive intent is actually the opposite of what you fear? Go back and take a closer look. The Rebel fears being overlooked or ignored. She eats to be accepted for who she is. The Fraud is afraid she's not good enough. She eats to feel more secure. See the connection? The positive intent of your eating behavior is actually a protection mechanism, with good feelings being the end goal.

Food for Thought

When I was going up and down the scale, jumping around my bedroom at eleven at night trying to work off the sins of indulgence from that day or the ones I anticipated for the next, I hated myself. I hated the part of me that made me engage in those out-of-control behaviors. I didn't understand them, and I hated myself for doing them. Maybe you feel similarly? Take comfort in knowing that underneath your behaviors, you're trying to take care of yourself. As crazy as it may sound, your intent is good.

Play around again with identifying the positive intent of your eating habits, but this time reframe your question. Close your eyes, and ask the objecting part of you, "What's my biggest fear?" Once you uncover the fear that drives you to overeat, see if the positive intent becomes clearer to you. Record any new insights in your weight-release journal.

Someone Who Tried This Before You

Julia was a dynamic, successful entrepreneur. Despite being barely five feet tall, she had a remarkable ability to take command of a room, projecting confidence and energy. Yet underneath her confident exterior she secretly felt inadequate, as though she were an interloper who would soon be found out to be operating by the seat of her pants. She came to see me because, although she was very successful in her professional life, she couldn't figure out how to control her weight. She'd recently ballooned and had gotten into a new habit of wearing crisp white shirts untucked to hide her expanding midsection.

After digging in, she realized that her overeating served to quell her fears of being found out as the Fraud. When we dug deeper, she discovered that the positive intent of her eating was to help her feel "big enough" for the business world and prove that she could keep up with the big boys' club that dominated her profession and often left her feeling inferior.

♥

Ava confessed to me in our first session together that she was consuming over 1,000 calories a day in alcohol; she was going through at least one bottle of wine a night, plus a cocktail or two. Her weight was up, and she wanted to make a change. That said, she didn't want to change her drinking habits! When we dug in and explored her objections to cutting back on the Cabernet, Ava uncovered a deep loneliness. A mother of three young children, she described a routine of running around all day, every day, in an effort to take care of her kids and maintain the household. Her primary personality type was that of the very common and socially accepted Giver. Every night after the dinner dishes were done and the kids were put to bed, she would pour herself a glass of wine, sit down in front of the computer, and pass the next several hours connecting with friends on Facebook or playing online games. She justified the activity as much-needed "me" time.

I completely agreed with her that she needed time to recharge from all her selfless giving, but she was going about it in a way that was unhealthful and potentially destructive. Yet, faced with the idea of giving up her after-dinner drinks, she broke down in tears. Together we realized how much she'd wrapped up her identity in her drinking. Her friends knew her as the fun, boozy after-hours mommy, and she worried that if she stopped drinking, she'd be less likable and people would no longer want to connect with her. Underneath the Giver was the Fraud. Ava suffered from deep feelings of loneliness and worthlessness. She feared that if she stopped drinking and were sober, her friends and family would see the real, "flawed," unlovable her and abandon her. The positive intent of her drinking was to feel worthy and loved.

If, after digging in yourself, what first comes to mind doesn't feel like the big revelation you were hoping for, chances are you just haven't dug deep enough. Let me give you an example of how to go deeper. Let's say you're a sucker for the office sweets. There's often leftover birthday cake in the break room, your favorite candy bar in the vending machine, or a bowl of Hershey's Kisses on a coworker's desk. Every afternoon, you find yourself grabbing a handful (more like a purse full, really!) and heading back to your office. When looking for the positive intent of your junk-food habit, all you come up with is that sweets are a reward; they give you a quick lift, and that feels good. It's as simple as that. Right? Not quite. Let's dig a little deeper.

In this scenario, imagine what you might have been feeling right before you decided you needed a lift. Rewind to the moment right before you thought of visiting the vending machine and play your thoughts back in s-l-o-w motion. Right before you thought of indulging in an afternoon candy bar, were you feeling happy, satisfied, content? More than likely, you weren't. In fact, you were probably feeling quite dissatisfied. Let's imagine that you were feeling exhausted and run down, and at the moment you realized you were feeling bad, candy seemed like the perfect fix because you knew from past experience that it'd instantly give you an energy boost. Not so fast! Before you jam that candy bar into your mouth, ask yourself, "What's *underneath* my feeling of exhaustion?" After giving it some thought, you answer, "I've been working like a dog and there's still more to be done and I'm afraid I won't get it all done in time." Good. Go deeper. If you can't get it all done, what would that mean about you? "I'm a failure. I'm not worthwhile. I'll get fired and end up destitute." Aha! There's the fear. On a deeper level, you're afraid of failing and ending up on skid row. Next, ask yourself, "What's the opposite of this fear? What would make me feel better and less afraid?" You answer, "I'll get the job done quickly and successfully, and that will make me feel accomplished and, ultimately, worthy." There it is—your positive intent for eating! In this scenario, you are the Overachieving Multitasker. You're using food as a release from all your relentless doing and to give you extra energy to do more. Ultimately, you crave feelings of accomplishment and self-worth.

Let's try another example. You ask yourself, "What is the positive intent of my unhealthful eating habits?" You determine that you overeat because it gives you something to do in social situations. Fair enough. You then ask yourself, "What feelings are underneath this behavior?" After giving it some thought, you determine that the energy in a crowded room makes you feel stifled and uncomfortable. Good. Keep going. You then realize that, in social situations like the one described, you feel overwhelmed—as though you can't handle everyone's "stuff." Bingo! You have a fear of being engulfed by other people's energy. Next, ask yourself, "What is the opposite of this fear of being overwhelmed? What would make me feel better?" Finally you come up with "I'd feel better if I were more insulated and relaxed." There it is, your positive intent. In this scenario, you are the Reluctant Mystic. You're using food to buffer yourself from the energy of those around you. Ultimately, you want to feel protected and grounded.

Are you beginning to understand that your positive intent for overeating is the opposite of what you fear? Let's look at one more example before moving on. Start by asking yourself, "What do I get out of overeating?" Let's say you determine that you overeat because you're bored. The next question to ask is "What feelings are underneath my boredom?" You determine that underneath the boredom are feelings of angst and dissatisfaction with your job. Good. Go deeper. Pinpoint the fear. What are you afraid of? You realize you're not pushing yourself to your highest potential because you're afraid that you might not be up to snuff and your best efforts might fail. Voilà—you're afraid that people will discover you're not good enough. Next, ask yourself, "What is the opposite of this fear? What would make me feel better?" You answer, "I'd feel better if I had the confidence and the courage to go after a career that might better fulfill me." There it is, your positive intent. In this scenario, you are the Fraud. You are using food to distract yourself from feelings of insecurity and unworthiness. Ultimately, you crave feelings of safety, confidence, and acceptance, and that's why you overeat.

In Weeks 3 and 4 of the Full-Filled program, I will teach you a strategy that helps you honor your positive intent in new, better ways that don't involve the break room birthday cake and give you the tools for confronting and releasing emotional pain. But before you can confront and release your fears, you must clearly identify them and, in turn, name the good feelings and positive experiences you truly want instead.

Dig In: Pinpoint Your Fear

Recall the first thing that came to your mind when you asked the objecting part of you, "What am I getting out of overeating and being overweight?" Then ask yourself, "What feelings of discontent are underneath this objection?" Dig deeper. Rewind to the moment right before you last thought of overeating and play your thoughts back in s-l-o-w motion. Imagine what you were feeling right before you decided to indulge. Identify any feelings of discontent and write them down. Then ask yourself, "What fear is underneath these feelings of discontent?" Write down your insights. Once you identify the fear, ask yourself, "What would make me feel less afraid? What would make me feel better?" The deeper you dig, the closer you will get to the positive intent—your true reason for overeating. Your positive intent will almost always turn out to be a basic want or need such as joy, peace, acceptance, worthiness, love, or contentment. When you get right down to it, we're all hungry for the same things.

Breaking the Cycle of Overeating

Now that you understand that you eat to avoid pain and feel good, let's take a look at where this cycle originated. In other words, when did you decide that food was the easiest go-to when you were craving good feelings? Think back to your childhood for a moment. At some point during your formative years, you more than likely experienced some emotional pain: a friend moving away, the loss of a pet, a bully at school, your parents' divorce. Whatever the pain was, it made you feel bad, and because you didn't like feeling bad (who does?), you looked for something that would make you feel good—not in a week or a month but right then and there. You got the idea from a family member, a friend, or all the kids eating fast food on TV that perhaps eating would make you feel better. Lacking a more constructive "adult" way to deal with your pain, you decided to give it a try and found that, at least temporarily, eating made you feel good, and very quickly. Great! You found an easy solution that quickly soothed your pain.

Except.

You soon discovered that if you'd eaten too much or eaten something you weren't "supposed" to eat, you felt physical pain, with a side of emotional guilt. The combination of physical pain and guilt made you feel bad again, and feeling bad made you feel, well, bad! Desiring to feel good again, you did what you knew worked. You ate, and once again you temporarily felt relieved. Only each time the temporary good feelings of food wore off, not only did you wrestle with nagging guilt, you were also faced with the same bad feelings that had gotten you eating in the first place! Though you'd hoped that food would rescue you from your pain, you discovered that your painful feelings never diminished; they simply held steady and waited for you to return. And the cycle of overeating continued.

Feel Bad → Eat → Feel Good → Feel Bad/Guilty → Eat

Exhausting, isn't it? And doomed to failure, as you know. I can't tell you how many clients have come to me utterly depleted and defeated by their efforts to break the cycle of overeating by not eating. Boy, can I relate to that one! Back when I was struggling with food, I tried starvation, deprivation, and obsessively counting calories. Ironclad willpower, the main ingredient of most popular diets, can carry you through for some time—weeks, months, even a year—yet at some point you feel emotional pain again, the kind you really hate to feel, and you break down and eat. Maybe you justify your actions by saying "Just this once won't matter" or, even more boldly, "If an extra-large pizza is what it takes to get me through this rough patch, so be it." Not only is this pattern exhausting, but breaking the cycle of overeating by trying not to eat is a strategy doomed to failure because it doesn't address the painful feelings you're trying to stuff down or massage with food. It's a temporary Band-Aid. That's all it is and all it will ever be.

So what will work?

First things first. Throwing a wrench into the cycle of overeating starts by reducing the sting of guilt. You can do this by simply acknowledging the positive intent of your eating, which is to make you feel good right now. If you can give yourself a break for wanting to feel good and for unconsciously going about it the wrong way, you'll save yourself a lot of painful guilt, which will, in turn, stave off more overeating. This guilt-neutralization strategy is a good one, especially for short-term relief. Ultimately, however, you must come face-to-face with the bad feelings—that is, the fear or pain that you're attempting to repress or massage with food. You need to name the good feelings and positive experiences you truly want instead (for example, feeling less exhausted at work so you feel more productive and confident). When you can name what you're truly hungry for, you've already won half the battle.

Someone Who Tried This Before You

Joyce was a successful social worker who routinely worked with divorce and custody battles and had struggled with her weight her entire life. She was 150 pounds over her "ideal" weight by the time she contacted me.

As we sought to resolve Joyce's internal conflict, she discovered the positive intent of her up-and-down weight gain. She told me that, throughout her early childhood, her mother had been emotionally unstable, prone to outbursts of screaming and crying. Those outbursts had terrified young Joyce, and she had taken comfort in the only thing available at the time: food.

Ironically, as an adult, Joyce got into a professional field where she was routinely around people in emotional crisis. She overate in reaction to the stress of the job. Her cycle looked like this: binge-ing and weight gain, followed by restrictive dieting and short-lived weight loss.

Soon after we began working together, Joyce discovered that her eating habits, as well as her extra weight, were a protection mechanism, a buffer between her and the often unstable external world. As Joyce looked for the positive intent, she realized that the part of her that drove her to overeat was trying to keep her safe and protected from a crazy mother and a crazy world. Once Joyce brought her adult understanding and compassion to her younger "abused" self, her urge to overeat began to diminish.

Resolve Your Internal Tug-of-War

Now that you understand that there is positive intent behind every morsel of food you put in your mouth, you may be thinking, "Okay. I get it. I eat to feel better about myself, yet I'm still miserable carry-ing around all this extra weight. I still feel stuck. Now what?"

I'm glad you asked. Understanding your motivation for eating is great awareness, but it typically won't create behavior change on its own. Before you can transform your current eating habits into new, healthful behaviors that will make you slim and healthy for a lifetime, you must take an important intermediate step. You will use your new awareness to start the transformative process of resolving your inner conflict.

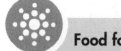

Food for Thought

No matter how much you eat or how unhealthy you are, you are trying to get something good out of your behaviors, or you wouldn't do them. Once you know the positive intent of any behavior, you will know what really matters to you and find better, positive, healthful ways to achieve that intent. I wonder what new, delightful ways your positive intent will be laced throughout your dream life as you progress through this program.

Take a moment now to acknowledge that the positive intent of your unhealthful eating habits is actually a gift that a part of you has been trying to give yourself for some time now. Whether it be the gift of comfort, safety, freedom, acceptance, or connection with others, a part of you has been working very hard to give those wonderful things to you. Sure, stuffing yourself until you make yourself sick hasn't been the best way to go about it, but your intention has been absolutely positive, a gift, really. A gift that a part of you who loves you wants you to have. This loving part of you has been trying persistently, loyally, and with uncompromising diligence and dedication to give it to you for years. Wow! I bet you didn't know that the part of you that gets you to sneak spoonfuls of chocolate frosting loved you so completely!

Next, I want you to take a moment and acknowledge the positive intent of the part of you who wants you to be slim. This may seem obvious—that the part of you who says "yes" to being slim wants something good for you. But really think about it for a moment. If you were slim and healthy, what would you also be? Appreciated? Happy? Fulfilled?

Both parts of you want something really good for you. That's wonderful! Can you recognize that love is at the heart of your internal conflict? And because both parts of you are armed with love, neither side will give up until it gets you what you truly, deeply desire.

It's a standoff in which, on any given day, one side of you is winning the battle. Maybe today, the slim and healthy part of you has the advantage. You're eating well, exercising regularly, and treating yourself kindly. Maybe you've even dropped a few pounds. But not for long. At some point, the other part of you, who's craving the deep gifts such as comfort, safety, and freedom (and who is not getting them), will tug back harder and stronger and regain the upper hand. Back into the cookie jar you'll go! What does this tug-of-war look like? Yo-yo dieting. Do you understand now why your struggle up and down the scale never seems to end? What if I told you that both parts of you could win—that you could resolve your internal tug-of-war and finally have everything you want and need?

Food for Thought

One part of you is pulling and tugging in one direction—"I want to be slim, I want to be fit, and I want to be healthy"—and the other part of you is pulling and tugging the other way—"I want comfort, I want downtime, I want to eat what I want when I want to!" You've got a great tug-of-war going on inside of you. If you're tired and feel depleted, no wonder! Think of all the energy you're expending on this fight. Imagine for a moment that instead of all that pulling and grunting, instead of all that division, each part of you released the rope and dropped the fight. Imagine peace. Imagine resolve. What would that be like for you?

Take a moment to relax and drop inside, then do the following mindful meditation, "Resolve Your Inner Conflict," inspired by the work of Dr. Robert Dee McDonald.

Mindful Meditation: Resolve Your Inner Conflict

Close your eyes, and imagine the two parts of you in conflict. There is the part of you who enthusiastically says *yes* to releasing weight and being slim, healthy, and attractive and the part of you who adamantly says *no*. These two parts of you have been in conflict for a long time, and the time has come to resolve the conflict, to create wholeness within you.

The *yes* and *no* parts both live within you, within your body. Notice where in your body the *yes* part of you lives (usually in your belly, chest, or heart). Allow the *yes* part of you to leave that part of your body and come to rest in your hand. Notice that when the *yes* part of you arrives in the open palm of your hand, it becomes a symbol or a word that represents the gift it's been trying to give you. Remember, this is a positive gift. Clearly identify in your mind the gift that now rests in your hand, and say what it is out loud. Take your time with this. For example, you might say, "I hold the gift of happiness. What a wonderful gift." Sincerely thank this part of you for loving you and working so hard to give you what you so deeply desire. Say, "Thank you for this gift—for wanting to give it to me."

Now turn your attention to the part of you that says *no* to releasing weight and to being slim, and notice where in your body this part of you has been living (usually in your belly, chest, or heart). Allow the *no* part of you to leave that part of your body and come to rest in your other hand. Notice that when the *no* part of you arrives in the open palm of your hand, it becomes a symbol or a word that represents the gift it's been trying to give you. Clearly identify in your mind the gift that now rests in your hand, and say what it is out loud. For example, you might say, "I hold the gift of protection. This is also a wonderful gift!" Take a moment to acknowledge the gift from this other part of you. Say, "Thank you for this gift—for wanting to give it to me."

Now ask the part of you who wants to be slim and healthy if it can understand and appreciate the positive gift of the part of you who overeats. Then ask the part of you who overeats, Can you understand and appreciate the gift from the part of me who wants to be slim and healthy? Can both parts of you understand and appreciate what the other has been so diligently working towards? In your mind's eye, slowly bring your two hands together. As the *yes* and *no* parts of you clasp hands, you share a mutual appreciation of each other's gifts.

For the first time, each part of you understands and appreciates the value of the other's gifts. How wonderful! Both parts of you, fueled by love, have desperately wanted you to have the gifts you so deeply desire. As each part appreciates the positive gift of the other, notice how good that feels. With this new understanding and compassion, both the *yes* and *no* parts of you can now unite at a deep soul level and create something new—a gift that combines happiness and protection and that is greater and more powerful than the sum of its parts. Where there were two gifts, now there is one; where there were two parts of you, now you are whole and complete and can accept this new gift into the deepest parts of your mind, body, and spirit, through the past, present, and future.

Clients often tell me that when they do this mindful meditation, they feel a significant shift inside. They feel more awake, aware, refreshed, and renewed. Maybe you feel it, too? When the *yes* and *no* parts of you can connect on the level of positive intent, acknowledge each other's gifts, and set a new intent to achieve what you truly and deeply desire in life, an amazing thing happens: you discover that you can finally, and significantly, change your behaviors and create the body and life of your dreams.

Someone Who Tried This Before You

With her warm smile and charismatic personality, Satia seemed as though she had it all together. She held a good job in finance and others envied her extreme discipline. After losing more than 60 pounds, she became a competitive bodybuilder to keep herself slim. To make weight for competition, she would endure starvation diets and hours of grueling workouts. Satia meticulously tracked everything she ate and swore off fat and carbohydrates for her muscle-building diet of skinless chicken breasts, canned tuna, and protein powder. Looking at her six-pack abs and bulging muscles, you would think she was the model of willpower and self-discipline. But that was only half the story.

When Satia wasn't good, she was very, very bad. She'd scarf down volumes of forbidden foods in record time. Because she binged when she was alone, no one knew her secret, and she worked hard to keep it that way. Shame and guilt were the fuel for her intense workouts and austere diet.

Satia had a raging inner conflict: part of her would do almost anything to be ultraslim and fit, but another part of her craved the release of the binge. The more she tried to control her inner binger, the worse her binges became.

Soon after working my program, Satia realized that there weren't good and bad parts of her; all parts of her wanted something truly good for her. She wanted to be slim, fit, and healthy and also to feel free of strict discipline and control. She was simply going about getting those things in unhealthful and opposing ways. Once Satia identified the gifts of freedom and health that she'd been trying to give herself, she was able to resolve her inner conflict and look for better and more effective ways to receive what she truly desired without the frequent bingeing.

How did she do it? She stopped restricting and controlling what she ate and allowed herself to eat what her body wanted. That provided her with the sense of freedom she so desperately craved. Most people who heavily restrict and control their eating behaviors fear that if they don't, they'll eat uncontrollably. But it's actually the restriction that causes the out-of-control behavior. Satia discovered that when she tuned into her body and let it tell her what it needed most, her eating habits slowly began to change. Soon she found herself preferring and therefore choosing healthful foods in appropriate amounts to fill her up. Eventually, her binge behavior completely disappeared.

Once you resolve your inner conflict, you'll find it surprisingly easy to create new ways to receive what you deeply want and need more fully than ever before—without the food! Does this mean you will instantly stop overeating? Nope. More than likely, you will eat the "wrong" things and too much of them from time to time. And guess what? That's exactly what I want you to do. Your future screw-ups are actually your ticket to success. Don't believe me? Then turn to the next week of the Full-Filled program for the surprising news that will change how you eat and think forevermore.

Progress Report

Over the next seven days, be sure to:

1. **Pinpoint your objection to becoming the person of your dreams.** Once you have a clear picture in your mind of the person you want to become, ask yourself, "Is there any part of me that objects to realizing this dream?" Notice any sensations of discomfort that come up. There are all sorts of objections you might have to becoming your dream self. Though the act of dreaming feels safe, to imagine really becoming that person can scare us. Write your insights down in your weight-release journal.

2. **Identify what you're getting out of your current eating habits and weight.** At the root of your unhealthful eating habits is something called "positive intent." Said a different way, you're getting something positive out of overeating and being overweight. There are all sorts of things you might be getting out of your eating habits and excess weight: protection, comfort, security, and approval, to name a few. Write your insights down in your weight-release journal.

3. **Uncover the fear that drives you to overeat.** Your positive intent is actually the opposite of what you fear, so ask yourself, "What's my biggest fear?" Dig deep. Rewind to the moment right before you last overate and play your thoughts back in s-l-o-w motion. Note the thoughts that precede the behaviors you want to change. Pinpoint the fear underneath your feelings of dissatisfaction and take note of it. Write your insights down in your weight-release journal.

4. **Accept the gift.** Acknowledge that the positive intent of your unhealthy eating habits is actually a gift that a part of you has been trying to give yourself for some time now. Whether it is the gift of comfort, safety, freedom, acceptance, or connection with others, a part of you has been working very hard to give those wonderful things to you for years. Sincerely thank that part of you for loving you and working so hard to give you what you so deeply desire.

5. **Resolve your inner conflict.** Before you can transform your current eating habits into new, healthful behaviors that will make you slim and healthy for a lifetime, you must resolve your inner conflict. Allow the part of you who says *yes* to losing weight and the part of you who adamantly says *no* to connect and acknowledge each other's gifts. Once both parts of you are united and whole, you can easily create the body and life of your dreams.

Your Slip-Ups Are the Keys to Your Success

What I'm about to tell you may surprise you, as it conflicts with the basic premise of most every other diet and weight loss plan. Are you ready for it?

In order to achieve long-lasting weight release, you must occasionally overeat.

Let me guess—you're not swallowing it, right? That's because most of us who overeat tend to see our eating habits in stark black-and-white terms. We are either eating "good" or totally screwing up, either succeeding or failing big time. There's no in between.

Not true.

Here's what is true: your belief that you must always be good and never overeat has prevented you from becoming slim and healthy for a lifetime. This is a departure from the mentality of most weight loss plans, which encourage strict discipline and absolute adherence to the "rules." But hear me out: black-and-white, all-or-nothing thinking is never going to get you anywhere. Except up and down the scale.

Thankfully, you can take another approach that *will* get you somewhere. It starts with the idea that there is no such thing as "blowing it." In fact, you must overeat in order to transform your unhealthful eating habits into new, healthful behaviors.

Hard to believe, isn't it? Let me explain. As you continue on your weight-release journey, you will make mistakes. You'll slip up. And I encourage you to do so because mistakes are excellent teachers; you can't learn without them. With that in mind, your success from this day forward will depend on your willingness to regard each mouth-stuffing episode, each sneaky bite of pie, as a learning experience that you will use to build the foundation for big-time behavior change.

In Week 3 of the Full-Filled program, you will learn to:
- Ditch the all-or-nothing approach to weight loss
- Self-correct and avoid the megabinge
- Make the DIF-ference for lasting success
- Begin to change your behaviors by simply changing how you think

Failure Is Just Feedback

Your progress will advance in exact proportion to how kind you are to yourself, so as you begin Week 3 of the Full-Filled program, **set your intention to be forgiving and kind to yourself as you allow yourself to learn from your slip-ups and mistakes**. Take a deep, cleansing breath and become present with your intention.

Before you get one more day into this program, you must accept the simple truth that you will overeat again. While you recently developed some new insight into what motivates you to overeat and weigh what you do, it doesn't mean that you're now immune to the afternoon snack attack. Sorry to disappoint you, but while you're discovering new and better ways to honor your positive intent—that is, satisfy your deep hunger—you will have days when the siren song of the vending machine pulls you right in and, before you know it, you'll be standing in the break room with an empty candy wrapper and a fistful of guilt. Relax.

Remember, the Full-Filled program is not about becoming a "good" versus a "bad" eater. There are no good and bad parts of you; all parts of you want something good for you. So instead of beating yourself up when a vending machine moment happens, you will chalk it up to a learning experience that is imperative to your transformative growth. In short, you'll neutralize the guilt and move on.

"Sure," you say. "Easier said than done."

Okay, maybe it doesn't sound so easy, but think for a moment about how a baby learns to walk. Before you took your first steps, you probably pulled yourself up off the ground only to plop back down hundreds of times. Did you think to yourself, "Oh, no, I've blown it. I'll never learn to walk because I never have up until now. I must be a defective baby"? No. You found the whole learning process irresistible and fun, and, most important, you kept at it. As a result, you eventually became a great walker.

Making mistakes is a natural part of everyone's learning process, so why is it that when it comes to our eating habits, we expect ourselves to get it right the first time? Or when we slip up and eat a whole cheesecake, we expect ourselves to miraculously stop overeating forever—even though we are armed with nothing other than guilt-inspired resolve? "I will never eat cheesecake again. In fact, I will never overeat again!" Such an expectation not only is unreasonable, it actually prevents you from making progress, chiefly because anything less than perfection, which is impossible, makes you feel like a failure.

As far as I'm concerned, you need to take that F-word out of your vocabulary. Feelings of failure make you feel bad, and you know what you do when you feel bad—you eat to feel better! On top of that, when you repeat the pattern over and over again, week after week, month after month, year after year, you inevitably lose faith in yourself—and that's the greatest crime of all.

When you can embrace the idea that there's no such thing as failure, only feedback, all of a sudden every slip-up becomes just that—a slip-up. Big deal. And just as a baby learns to walk by standing up and tumbling to the floor and standing up again and again, you, too, will get up after every fall until being slim and healthy for a lifetime is as easy as a stroll through the park.

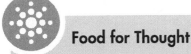

Food for Thought

If you were perfect, you wouldn't be human; you wouldn't be alive—because everything that's alive is constantly learning, changing, and growing. So forget about perfection; it ain't going to happen. Plus, what if it's your imperfections, your humanity, that make you lovable? Chew on that one.

Self-Correcting Is Key

So you slip up. You eat a few bites too many at dinner or snack in the middle of the day when you're not truly hungry, and that's okay. What about the megabinges that get you into big trouble— the I've-already-blown-it-I-might-as-well-go-*all*-the-way eating episodes? Are those okay, too? Before I answer that, let's look at how a megabinge often plays out. It goes something like this: You've been on a healthful eating streak for the past few weeks. You feel confident and energetic, and you're elated each morning by how your clothes are fitting. "Eating 'good' is easy," you think. "I can totally stay on track and finally lose the weight I've gained over the past year."

But then the weekend rolls around, and you find yourself at a big social event. After indulging in a cocktail or two and catching up with friends, you pass the dessert table and notice a delicious-looking cheesecake. You decide to take just one bite (cheesecake is your favorite, after all), but instead of putting the fork down after one bite, you proceed to eat the entire piece. And since you ate the cheesecake, why not try the chocolate dessert and whatever else you find?

After this major indulgence, you go home and eat more. Again, you already blew it, you reason, so you might as well go all the way. Of course, after you let this one slip throw you into a full-on binge, you're left frustrated and defeated, convinced that "Nothing works for me because nothing has ever worked for me" or "I'll never change because I've never been able to change" or "I always do this." You sink into food despair, and before you know it, you're eating more to numb the painful feelings of overeating. Have you ever had an experience like this? It feels pretty awful, doesn't it?

To stop a minor slip-up from throwing you into a regrettable tailspin, you will use one of my favorite weight-release techniques: self-correction. Consider this: an airplane that flies from San Francisco to New York never flies in a single straight line because, in actuality, it cannot. Due to wind currents, other weather conditions, and a number of other factors, a plane from SFO to JFK is constantly being thrown off course, so the plane's navigation system continuously self-corrects. Think about it: when a plane hits turbulence that knocks it off course, the pilot doesn't continue to fly in the wrong direction, does she? Nor does she land the plane because she "messed up." No. She makes adjustments and corrections to get back on course and continue towards her destination. Because life, like unexpected turbulence, can often throw your eating habits off course, you will apply the same self-correction technique to your weight-release strategy.

Food for Thought

Perhaps the most important shift that you will make in this program is the shift from condemning yourself for your slip-ups and throwing up your hands in defeat to recognizing that your mistakes are actually doorways to your dream future.

Take a quick inventory: how long does it regularly take you to get back into balance and back on track after a minor slip-up or a major indulgence? Days? Months? Years? What if it took you only twenty-four hours or less to get back on track and motivated towards your weight-release goals? What if after just one bite too many, you automatically put the fork down? That would feel pretty good, wouldn't it? I have clients who have learned how to self-correct from meal to meal and even bite to bite, and guess what? They no longer struggle with their weight.

When you correct your course after you have strayed only slightly, you'll feel better about yourself, you'll feel better in your body, and you'll be amazed how much less frequently you slip into the I've-already-blown-it-I-might-as-well-go-*all*-the-way mind-set.

Stay the Course

For self-correction to work, you must wait until after you've over-eaten to apply this practice. *After* is key. Most of us try to prevent overeating at the height of a craving by resisting the first bite. That's like trying to make a U-turn in an eighteen-wheeler truck that's bar-reling down the highway at eighty miles per hour. It's not going to happen safely. Overeating is no different. Trying to stop midway from hand to mouth when your craving is at its climax requires an enormous amount of energy and willpower. Not only that, it rarely works, which leads to more feelings of frustration and failure, and you know what feelings of failure trigger? That's right—more over-eating. My advice: don't try to turn a binge into a teachable moment. If you feel a fierce craving coming on—bring it on! Let it happen, and resolve to enjoy your food while you're eating it. If afterward you feel that you've overdone it, you'll self-correct then.

Take a few moments to revisit the memory of the last time you overate. What emotions came up after you stuffed yourself way past full? Disappointment? Frustration? Guilt? Defeat? Negatively charged emotions such as those throw your energy off-balance, and when you're out of balance—energetically, emotionally, spiritually, or physically—you feel bad, which will eventually lead you back to the food.

Self-correction, then, is what you do to return to a feel-good, balanced state after you've been thrown off course so you don't go to the dark place (and by dark I mean the cupboard). It's only when you're feeling renewed and good about yourself that you can truly honor your positive intent—that is, get the good feelings you crave on a deeper level, such as comfort, safety, and joy, without diving into the five-pound bag of chips.

Food for Thought

Long-term maintenance is nothing more than self-correcting within twenty-four hours or less. So the more you practice and master self-correcting, the more stable your slim weight will become. Imagine what it would be like if the first 2 pounds you gained were always the first 2 pounds you released. Seriously, imagine that right now.

Below are three levels of self-correcting techniques to rebalance and renew your energy and return you to a feel-good, positive state after an overeating episode. If you find yourself resisting the process (wallowing in despair can seem so appealing at times), it may be that you simply aren't used to treating yourself well. If you routinely put self-care at the bottom of your priority list, under your career, family, friends, even your pets, take a moment now and think about the last time you were on a plane. What do the flight attendants always tell you to do? They tell you that in an emergency situation, you must put your own oxygen mask on first before helping anyone else. That isn't a moral commentary. It is a rule of survival. The only way you can really take good care of others is by first taking care of yourself.

LEVEL ONE: RENEW ON YOUR OWN—EVERY DAY
The self-correcting tools in this level are fairly quick and easy things you can do on your own to rebalance yourself energetically,

emotionally, spiritually, and physically to get back on track to feeling good. They include working out, meditating, getting a good night's rest, hydrating, eating a healthful breakfast, or simply running an inner dialogue that's positive, gentle, and accepting. The key to these activities is that they leave you feeling renewed and better about yourself and your body than when you started. Try any one of these, which are my and my clients' favorites.

- **Meditate.** A few minutes of quiet time, focusing on your breath, can do wonders to calm and center you. Try this simple meditation. Visualize a beautiful white light of renewing energy that you breathe deep into your lungs. Feel this positive energy spread from your lungs into your bloodstream, and let your heart gently pump it throughout your body, from the top of your head to the tips of your toes to the back of your mind. With each exhalation, release any concerns, fears, tension, worries, or tightness. Imagine them flowing down into the earth, where they are composted into fresh, fertile soil. When your mind wanders, as it often will, simply bring your attention back to your breath. Start with five minutes and work your way up to twenty. This simple meditation will help center and renew you.

- **Make a Feel-Good List.** In your weight-release journal, list all the things that you're grateful for in your life and everything that makes you feel good. These could be very small things, such as the sun shining on your face or receiving a smile from a stranger. The key is that everything you list makes you feel really good. After you write them down, spend a few moments enjoying your favorites as you revisit them in your mind. If you're reading this and thinking, "That's too simple," just stop and try it. Making a Feel-Good List is extremely powerful and has been proven to have a long-lasting effect on your state of mind. And a positive state of mind positively affects your eating behaviors.

- **Exercise.** Nothing beats an endorphin high and a good sweat to counteract an overeating episode and bring you back into feel-good balance. Think of exercise as something you do as a treat for yourself, rather than as punishment.

- **Restore.** Take time off to do something restorative, such as sinking into a hot bath. Alternatively, try a soak in the hot tub at your gym if you belong to one or a longer-than-usual hot shower if you don't. This is a simple but decadent activity that most of us don't take time to do.
- **Enjoy nature.** Spending time outside or taking a walk, especially in natural settings close to trees, plants, or water, can be enormously renewing and rebalancing.
- **Listen to music.** Let your favorite tunes take you to a positive place where you can calm down and fill up on positive energy. If you don't play music at home, begin to. If you commute by bus or train, make using your MP3 player a daily habit.
- **Enjoy your pet.** Spend some quality time with your or a friend's pet. Let his or her gentle spirit bring you back to your center.
- **Say affirmations.** Crank up your inner iPod with feel-good messages, such as "I am whole" and "All is well." Did you know that when you're feeling low, you're often just one thought away from feeling better? Introducing affirmative thoughts into your life is a quick, easy tool that really works. Remember, people around you cannot hear your inner playlist!
- **Sleep.** Did you know that losing sleep boosts cravings and encourages weight gain? Sleep deprivation also messes with your mood, so prioritize your nightly visit to dreamland. Catching up on your Zs may be just the ticket to feeling refreshed and renewed.
- **Play.** Engage in a favorite hobby, such as creating art, making jewelry, knitting, or gardening. Play renews the spirit like nothing else.

Because Level One self-correcting tools are fairly quick and easy, I recommend that in addition to using them to return you to a feel-good, positive state after an overeating episode, you practice them daily. When you dedicate just ten minutes a day to these renewal practices, you will soon discover that you are less likely to slip up and overeat in the first place! By putting yourself into a feel-good state every day, you prevent overeating. Two benefits for the price of one!

Food for Thought

We all lead busy lives, so it can seem difficult to fit in self-correction and self-renewal, which is why it's so important to put self-correction practices into place that are quick, easy, and extremely effective. Use simple renewal practices that will take you only five or ten minutes a day to do. I promise, their benefits will dramatically outweigh your time investment. Whenever someone tells me she doesn't have enough time for these practices, I know she is really saying that self-care is not a priority. Make it a priority! You will soon find that the few minutes you invest in self-renewal will become a comforting ritual, and they will also work wonders on your self-confidence and success.

Think about it: what is it you like to do that brings you pleasure and gives you energy and inspiration? Ask yourself at the beginning of each day, "What can I do to renew myself today to honor my positive intent—my deep emotional hunger? What can I do that will provide me with a sense of comfort, safety, and joy?" Even if it's as simple as listening to your favorite music on your way to work, make sure you do something. Remember, all I'm talking about is ten minutes a day set aside for the purpose of making you feel good. You can find ten minutes in your day in exchange for slim and healthy forever, can't you?

LEVEL TWO: RENEW WITH OTHERS

When you need a boost beyond Level One techniques to rebalance and renew your energy and put you back into a feel-good state after overeating, reach out to another person for support. Connect with your friends or your weight-release buddies, or simply put yourself into a social atmosphere where you feel inspired or encouraged by those around you. Have you created a weight loss support group or designated a support buddy yet? Having at least one person to connect with and share your progress with along the way will dramatically accelerate your progress, so if you have not yet reached out to an individual or a group, I strongly suggest you do so. I promise, you will be happy you did.

Level Two renewal techniques go beyond what you can accomplish on your own and draw on the positive energy and presence of another person or persons who can help you get back into a feel-good place after overeating. Try any of the following favorites of mine and my clients:

- Talk to a trusted friend. A ten-minute phone call to a buddy can be very restorative.
- Attend a yoga class, dance class, or group exercise class that you enjoy.
- Check in with your online or offline support group.
- Go to a worship service or engage in a spiritual practice, such as group prayer or meditation. Fill up on the positive energy that abounds in those settings.
- Go to an inspiring lecture, movie, or art gallery opening with a friend or group of like-minded people with whom you can engage in lively and renewing conversation.
- Laugh. Laughter is healing, restorative, and fun. In fact, laughing at our struggles is a great way to begin the transformative process. Tune in to your favorite comedy show, hang out with your funniest friend, or visit a comedy club.

LEVEL THREE:
RENEW WITH THE HELP OF A PROFESSIONAL

If you've practiced using both Level One and Level Two techniques to renew your feel-good energy after an overeating episode or a full-on binge, and after a couple of weeks you're still feeling out of balance and out of control, it's essential to consider the help of a trained professional, such as a traditional doctor, life coach, hypnotherapist, psychotherapist, counselor, or spiritual mentor. Why? If Level One and Level Two tools fail to get you back on track, the chances are high that you're in a really low-down funk. When you're in such a state, you may have difficulty putting your situation into perspective. A professional may be able to suggest a solution that has evaded you or simply guide you back to feeling good. In either case, a session or two with the right professional may be all that you need.

When choosing a professional, ask your friends and colleagues for recommendations and consult with your health care provider. Create a list of nearby recommended professionals, and conduct a series of interviews. Look for someone with a positive focus who makes you feel good about yourself, and then let your intuition be your guide. In addition to seeking traditional medicine, be open to alternative avenues, such as the help of a hypnotherapist, life coach, counselor, therapist, bodyworker, or spiritual adviser. Also consider attending a meditative retreat or holistic spa to renew your energy and your spirit.

Dig In: Get into Balance

In your Full-Filled Weight-Release Journal, make a list of which Level One self-correction tools will renew you on a daily basis and honor your positive intent. They should be things that you can do on your own for ten minutes every day. As you begin to integrate them into your daily routine, notice which ones are particularly effective at helping you rebalance after an overeating episode and putting you back into a state in which you feel good.

For example, a client of mine renews by paddling solo in her kayak. Another takes in the crashing waves at a nearby beach. Another gets back into a feel-good state by hitting the heavy bag at her gym.

Next, list the Level Two self-correction tools that will help you get back on course. Those are things you do with friends or your weight-release buddy. For example, some of my clients take a gardening class with a friend. Others sign up for ballroom, Zumba, or salsa lessons. Others enjoy hiking in nature with a trusted confidante or working out with a buddy at a gym. Joining a book club of like-minded readers is also a great Level Two self-correction tool.

Last, even though you may not know yet whether you will need the help of a professional, prepare yourself by identifying a trained professional whose help you will seek in the event that you need Level Three support. If you don't have someone in mind already, note the specific steps you will take to find someone, such as asking friends, colleagues, or your health care provider for recommendations and referrals.

Not only do your self-correction tools help you bounce back from an overeating episode, they send a powerful, positive message to your subconscious: *I am important. And I deserve to feel good.* They nourish you on a deep, spiritual level and, when practiced daily, keep your feel-good reservoir full. This is very important. When your underlying state of emotional and spiritual health is continuously replenished and nourished, you create what I call a Renewal Reserve. Self-correcting on a daily basis renews your reserves, enabling you to draw on them in times of stress and need, much like an emergency savings account. Think about it: when are you most likely to overeat? When you're feeling relaxed and renewed or run down? I bet you're much more likely to overdo it at the drive-through when your inner reserves are depleted. For that reason, I strongly encourage you to make your Level One self-correction tools a daily practice.

Someone Who Tried This Before You

Elizabeth was in her midfifties and had struggled with her weight for nearly forty years. She recalled that friends joked that she was like a walking yellow pages of weight loss programs, having tried them all over the years. When she came to me, she'd been caught in the same cycle of overeating for decades. She would eat a small, unsatisfying breakfast every morning, and without fail, by eleven o'clock she was ravenous. Since the food she kept in the house was not interesting to her, she'd drive to the nearest convenience store and load up on junk food. She'd eat it all in a frenzy, often in her car, and then return to her home office full of guilt. When dinnertime rolled around, she'd still be stuffed from her noontime binge and equally stuffed with self-loathing, so she would skip dinner. The next morning, she'd eat a teeny-tiny breakfast, and by midmorning, hungry again, she'd repeat her cycle of junk-food bingeing all over again.

We brainstormed about what might bring her back into balance after these episodes. How could she self-correct? After giving it some thought, Elizabeth realized that if she were to simply start her day with a good protein-rich breakfast, she'd set herself up for success all day long. Eating a better breakfast may seem like an obvious fix to you, but Elizabeth had gotten herself into such an automatic pattern of deprivation, followed by overindulging, that a simple tweak like this had eluded her.

She found that when she made this adjustment to her morning routine, she was never more than twenty-four hours away from getting back on course and motivated again towards her weight-release goals. Eating a protein-rich breakfast became a cornerstone self-correcting ritual in her life, and she has easily maintained it for over a year.

Allow me to be frank: becoming slim and healthy is not something bestowed on the worthy or a prize you win in the genetic lottery. Rather, it's a way of life. Every single person on the planet who is slim and healthy is so because he or she does things every day, as a matter of course, to be that way. Slim and healthy people choose foods that nourish them. They eat quantities that make their bodies feel great over time, and they exercise to feel vital and energized today, not three months in the future. Despite what you've learned from other diet and weight loss programs, reliable, long-lasting weight release is not an act of omission, meaning it's not what you cut out of your life that determines your success. Quite the opposite, really. Your eventual success will hinge on what you add to your life on a daily basis. When you eat nourishing foods, make time for exercise, get the right amount of sleep, and engage in self-care activities that make you feel good about yourself every day, long-lasting weight loss happens naturally.

So instead of giving yourself a drop-dead date to lose two dress sizes and reach that magic number on the scale, concentrate on the practices you will do every day that will replenish and renew you and will promote the slim and healthful lifestyle you want. Renewing requires that you be aware of how you are feeling physically, emotionally, and spiritually, so make a habit of checking in with how you're feeling every day. Consider creating "pause points" throughout your day when you pause and ask yourself, "How am I feeling? What would renew me right now?" Get into the habit of replenishing and renewing your reserves on a daily basis. When you're in balance and feeling good, you're less likely to turn to food to fill you up emotionally and spiritually.

Food for Thought

If you don't have renewal practices in place that you do every day, I'm not surprised that you've struggled with your weight, because in order for you to be slim and healthy, you have to put yourself first. You have to make yourself a priority. This is so important. If you don't know how to rebalance, how to renew yourself, how will you get back on track? If you do know how to renew, if you use the Level One, Level Two, and Level Three self-correction techniques, imagine how easy it will be for you to continually rebalance and progress and to feel and look better with each passing day.

Most spiritual and religious people will tell you that they spend a dedicated amount of time each day in quiet reflection or reading a prayer book. Why do they do it? Not for overnight redemption or because they're on the fast track to enlightenment. No, they devote a portion of every day to their faith because they are on an ongoing path towards greater spiritual fulfillment. That is how I want you to approach your weight-release journey. Get into the mind-set that you're on a path towards slim and healthful as a way of life. Though long-term towards motivation has great value (remember Liane's long-term motivation to walk a block and a half uphill?), daily short-term motivators that make you feel as good as possible all day, every day, are equally important. In the days and weeks ahead, begin to think of releasing weight more as a daily practice that brings its own rewards and less as a goal to be achieved in the distant future. You'll be surprised at how quickly the pounds take care of themselves.

Someone Who Tried This Before You

Stacy had a demanding job and regularly put in ten-hour days at the office. She'd come home, eat dinner, and then immediately retreat to her home office, where she'd jump back onto the computer. Without fail, within ten or fifteen minutes, she'd start craving food. She would find something she could snack on while she worked and would continue working and munching away late into the night.

After she described her routine to me, I asked her, "So when is your downtime?"

She joked, "Downtime? What's that? I don't have time for that."

"So you never give yourself downtime?" I asked.

"Do you think I need some?" she replied.

"What's the positive intent of your evening eating?" I asked.

Stacy thought for a moment and then replied that eating was the only way she could get through her work session after dinner.

"So eating gives you a bit of a break from the work?" I asked.

"Yes, it does," she realized.

An Overachieving Multitasker, Stacy treated eating as her mini-downtime, an emergency escape valve and her break from the pressure she put on herself to constantly be productive. Once she stopped beating herself up and let go of her demand to always be doing, doing, doing, she was able to allow herself to really relax. Instead of taking a break with a bowl of munchies while trying to push through a few more items on her endless "should-do" list, she was able to truly relax in a way she enjoyed: reading a book or magazine or zoning out in front of the TV.

Once Stacy started giving herself permission to relax on a daily basis, she not only found that she was eating less and enjoying her evening more, she also found that she was more productive at work because she started the day feeling more refreshed and renewed. Taking a break became Stacy's daily renewal practice, and as a result her true hunger—to feel accomplished, successful, and, ultimately, worthy—was eventually satisfied.

When you rely on your self-correction techniques, small slips into the snack bowl will become even smaller over time. Plus, the more you renew on a daily basis, even with simple indulgences such as solving a sudoku puzzle or checking in with a girlfriend over the phone, the more you will be able to handle the bigger stresses in life without turning to food. You will notice, too, that the faster you renew and bring yourself back into balance, the fewer cravings you'll have altogether and the less susceptible you will be to giving in to them. In fact, food will begin to fade into the background, because renewal techniques that make you feel good and honor your positive intent will become your new craving. You will know that you're making significant progress when you can self-correct in less and less time and more automatically. Your ability to get back on course may go from years to months to weeks to days to hours to minutes. You'll become like my client Delia, who, at her three-month review session, realized that she really didn't overeat anymore.

Food for Thought

From now on, I want your energy and enthusiasm to be focused on how quickly you can bring yourself back into balance after overeating. In order to do this, you will use the powerful tools presented in this program to heal the deep causes of your cravings, and you'll use your favorite renewing activities, such as listening to music or taking a walk in nature. This is the key to becoming slim and healthy forever. It is self-correcting.

Making the DIF-ference

Most of us measure our weight-release success one way—through pounds released. Unfortunately, and as you probably know, the scale doesn't always cooperate; it can be supremely misleading. Due to hormones, stress, water retention, sleep, and other factors, our weight fluctuates from day to day. Plus, the number on the scale is typically emotionally charged; it can send us into a tailspin of self-loathing if our weight creeps up even a half pound, shooting us straight back to our old "feel better" go-to: food. Given all this, it's important that you find ways to notice and document your progress off the scale.

Just as a plane flying from San Francisco to New York never flies in a single straight line, your progress will not happen in a straight line, either. You will improve, then slip, then self-correct, and then be more successful the next time around. If you demand of yourself only perfection, you will quickly become discouraged, because growth doesn't happen in a straight line.

Top athletes know this well. They have days when they are strong and at the top of their game and days when they feel wobbly. Wobbly, weak days are part of your progress, so don't waste your precious energy beating yourself up for having them. Instead, focus on a trend of improvement rather than ceaseless perfection. Remember the old adage "Two steps forward, one step back"? You may not have realized that the one step (and sometimes two or three) back actually makes possible the two steps (or four or five) forward.

 Food for Thought

Make small incremental changes continuously, even if they just involve increased awareness. Breakthroughs happen, too, as delightful bonuses, but real, lasting recovery comes in cultivating and appreciating the small steps forward. Let those small steps loom large in your awareness. Together, those small steps will create beacons of light that will brighten every aspect of your life if you simply allow them to happen.

One way to really notice if you are creating a slimming trend in your life is by tracking the DIF-ference you are making. DIF stands for:

Duration: *How long each overeating episode lasts*

Intensity: *How much and how quickly you eat during the episode*

Frequency: *How often your overeating episodes occur*

You can track a slimming trend by first becoming aware of how long, how much, and how often you overeat. **Duration** refers to how long an overeating episode lasts. Take a minute and think about your general eating habits. Do an extra few bites of cake at the office birthday party, for example, trigger you to eat "badly" the rest of the day, or do those bites turn into a full week of unhealthful eating choices? Perhaps for you, a few extra bites are as far as you go when your cravings are high. Others might let a few extra bites of cake turn into another piece or two eaten in rapid succession. How much and how quickly you eat during an overeating episode indicates **intensity**. And becoming aware of how often you let the office birthday cake throw you into a graze craze or a full-on binge is how you measure **frequency**.

Now that you understand the principle of self-correcting and have begun practicing some of the ways you can bring yourself back into balance after an overeating episode, set a new goal to reduce your DIF. Notice I said reduce, not eliminate. As I said before, you will overeat again. The problem is not occasional overeating. The problem is when small slips become long slides into overeating—episodes that last for days, weeks, or even months. If you simply self-correct when you have strayed only slightly and make the DIF-ference, so to speak, you will notice that the occasional slip-up has no lasting consequences to your body and weight. In fact, reducing your DIF will allow your weight release to happen more easily than it ever has before.

To reduce your DIF, you must first figure out where you are now so that you can appreciate the wonderful progress that you will make over time. In the Dig In exercise below, you will document the duration, intensity, and frequency of your most recent overeating episodes. Remember to catalog your answers in your Full-Filled Weight-Release Journal so that you can refer back to and track your progress over time.

 Dig In: Duration, Intensity, Frequency

Duration: How Long Do I Overeat For?

Ask yourself, "What is the duration of my usual overeating episode?" Does it last for two minutes? Two hours? Two days? Maybe you have a pattern of two weeks of "good" eating, followed by a week of "bad" choices. Document whatever your pattern is. If you have a hard time identifying a "usual," think of the last time you overate. How long did it last? Write it down.

_____

_____

_____

_____

Intensity: How Much Do I Overeat?

Now ask yourself, "What's the intensity? How much am I overeating?" Be specific: Are we talking about a couple extra bites of a sandwich after you're already feeling full or a whole extra plate, bag, or box of food? How many extra calories are you taking in? Do you eat until you feel just satisfied or until you feel immobile or even sick?

_____

_____

_____

_____

Frequency: How Often Do I Overeat?

Finally, ask yourself, "What's the frequency? How often am I overeating?" Is it many times a day because you graze, taking mindless handfuls here and there? Once a day? Once a week? Once a month?

_____

_____

_____

_____

After you've determined the general duration, intensity, and frequency of your overeating episodes, set one reasonable goal for reducing your DIF from this day forward. For example, if you tend to overeat at every meal, maybe you set your mind to reduce the frequency with which you overeat. Strive to overeat only once or even twice a day, and eat just the right amount the rest of the day. Once you achieve that goal, add in another. Don't try to reduce everything at once. That's where our ambitious minds love to go, but I'll say it again: the all-or-nothing approach only sets you up to fail, and I want you to notice real, identifiable improvement.

Track your progress in your Full-Filled Weight-Release Journal. Check back in every week, and take note of your DIF. Notice how your overeating has changed during that period. Are you overeating less? Do you overeat on healthier foods? Do you go for longer and longer stretches of eating well because you're renewing yourself daily?

Someone Who Tried This Before You

Camilla, a stay-at-home mother of two small kids and an extremely active volunteer, led a busy life. When she started following my program, she'd been struggling with her weight for over thirty years. She made great progress over the first few weeks of the program, but when she came to see me two months later, I noticed a hint of defeat in her voice. I asked her how she was doing.

"Terrible," she said. "I had been doing so well until this week, and I've already binged several times. I have no idea what's going on. I've thought so much about it and tried to get back to that good place, but I just can't. I feel like such a failure."

"Tell me, Camilla. What was different about these episodes from previous overeating episodes?"

She had to think for a moment. "The foods were different," she offered.

"Good," I replied. "How so?"

"Oh, the food was healthier than before, less junk."

"Anything else different? Did the episodes last as long as before? Did you eat as much?" I inquired.

"Well, no," she said. "They were shorter. In the past, I would have binged all day, but this time I just finished the package of whatever it was. The binges didn't outlast the morning."

"And did you eat the same amount of food as before?"

"No, actually, it was much less than before."

"So it seems like you aren't as good an overeater as you used to be?"

Camilla laughed. "I never thought of it that way."

"And before this program, how long had you ever gone binge-free?"

"The longest was a day or less."

"And how long was it this time?"

"Nine weeks."

"You just went your longest ever without binge eating, and when you did binge again, your binges were a pale imitation of your former efforts. And this is failure for you? Congratulations!"

Camilla began to perk up as she realized that perhaps this wasn't the end of her progress but actually an important step forward. She had learned how to overeat responsibly, one of the clearest indications of increased stability around food.

Like Camilla, you need to give yourself credit for your progress along the way, however inconsequential it may seem to be. This is crucial. When you focus on reducing the duration, intensity, and frequency of your overeating episodes, you will discover that incremental progress is your new goal. For example, you may overeat for a shorter amount of time, you may eat less, or you may even surprise yourself with out-of-the-blue cravings for healthful foods and indifference to some of your old guilty pleasures.

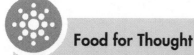

One of the keys to making significant changes to your behaviors is to notice and appreciate the new behaviors while they are forming. If you don't recognize that you are in a transition period in which you're learning and improving, you run the risk of giving up just when you are on the brink of lasting, permanent change. Make a priority of noting your small steps forward in your Full-Filled Weight-Release Journal.

The Mental Movie

Now you understand: improvement happens by self-correcting, not perfecting. Next, I want to teach you an especially powerful way to accelerate your progress. This self-correction technique will subtly, but surely, reshape your mind in a way that will influence a change in your eating behaviors. I call it the Re-Do, and it's a simple visualization process.

Whenever you simply imagine behaving the way you want to behave, new habits start to take root in your brain. It might sound like science fiction, but it's true. Research shows that each time you rehearse a new behavior, either in real life or in your mind (such as putting down your fork when you just start to feel full), your subconscious mind begins a rewiring process that influences a change in how you actually behave. In simple terms, you can imagine your way to new, healthful habits. It is a crucial step.

Let me give you an example of how this works: Jack Nicklaus, who was the golfer to beat before Tiger Woods hit the scene, was asked, "How do you do it, Jack? You are so perfect; do you ever make a mistake?" He answered, "Well, of course I make mistakes. I make them all the time. But what I do when I make a mistake is something that a lot of people don't do. When I hit a shot that doesn't go where I want it to go, I imagine hitting that shot again so that it goes just right. In my mind's eye, I hit the sweet spot and see the ball going exactly where I want it to go. I do this every time."

Sports psychologists and coaches have long understood the power of visualizing success in enhancing athletic performance. You can use the same technique of visualization to help you change your day-to-day behaviors around food. Research has shown that the brain does not know the difference between something that you vividly imagine and something you actually do.

Here's an example: In one study, some subjects were asked to vividly imagine playing the violin, while another group actually played the violin. As expected, the group that played showed changes in the motor cortex region of the brain, meaning that the nerve cells showed that they were physically playing the violin, bowing and fingering to create the sounds. Surprisingly, the researchers found that the motor cortexes of the group that only imagined playing the violin changed *in the same way*. They reflected the same activities. Sharon Begley, a *Wall Street Journal* columnist and the coauthor of *The Mind and the Brain: Neuroplasticity and the Power of Mental Force*, explains, "Merely thinking about moving produces brain changes comparable to those triggered by actually moving . . . the brain remakes itself based on something much more ephemeral than what we do. It rewires itself based on what we think."

 Food for Thought

Habits create neural pathways in the brain that, like well-worn trails, entice you to travel them again and again. Your eating behavior is like this. Each time you repeat the same behavior with the same thought patterns, you travel the path another time. The good news is that just as a new, better hiking trail can be created, so can new, more rewarding neural pathways.

If you simply imagine behaving the way you want to behave,

you will be creating your new trail. And each time you behave this new way, either in real life or in your mind, you make your new neural pathway more and more entrenched and easier to follow.

Want to give it a try? Let's say you recently overate and you're feeling bad about it. By re-doing your past slip-up in your mind, you start the process of replacing your previous behavior pattern with a new desired one.

Dig In: The Re-Do

- Think of the most recent situation when you overate.
- Imagine what feeling state you would like to have had during that situation. Remember your positive intent. What good feelings do you crave? To feel comforted? Worthy? Secure? Relaxed? Imagine feeling that way now.
- Imagine yourself feeling good in a similar eating situation in the future, and then visualize yourself behaving as you would like to in that situation.
- Feel the good feelings of behaving in this new way.
- Imagine a blank screen. This is an important step! This will signal to your mind that you have finished a complete behavior pattern. The subconscious needs to know clearly when the new behavior starts and when it finishes so that it can accept, and later "run," the new pattern in real life.
- Repeat the imagery three more times; the more you practice a behavior in your mind, the easier the new behavior will be to actualize in real life.
- Adjust your "mental movie" until you get it just the way you want it. Let it play a few times in your mind.

You can quickly reinforce your new imagined behavior by rehearsing it many times in your mind and feeling the positive feelings associated with doing it. For example, maybe you ate three doughnuts at work yesterday, and today you're regretting it. Ask yourself, "How could I behave differently next time? How do I want to behave differently next time?" Maybe you wish you'd only taken one bite or eaten carrot sticks or something more healthful instead. Whatever the case, think about the feel-good state that goes along with your desired behavior, and then imagine yourself feeling that way and behaving differently in the future.

It's important that when you re-do, you really focus on associating a positive feeling with the imagined behavior. Emotionally charged behaviors, both good and bad, stick in our subconscious, so if you imagine choosing carrots over doughnuts, let yourself feel the positive charge associated with making that choice. Imagine how good your body feels when nourished by healthful food. Then, the next time someone brings doughnuts into the office, your mind will remember the positive feelings associated with passing on the doughnuts and eating carrots instead. Before you know it, you've passed up the raised and glazed. You discover that your imagined behaviors have influenced and become your actual behaviors! Pretty amazing, right? Think of your Re-Do as a working draft for your new eating habits. As counterintuitive as it sounds, I encourage you to give it a try. You'll be pleasantly surprised that when you rewrite your past, you rewrite your future.

Food for Thought

Ask yourself, "How could I behave differently next time? How could I behave *better* next time?" Life offers us the same situation over and over again, until we figure out how to best deal with it. It's as if we get infinite practice opportunities until we get it right, and then we move on. So when you slip up and overeat, ask yourself, "What is there to learn here?" These are the questions of a learning mind, one focused on continuous improvement. These are the questions that will advance you.

Timing Is Everything

The best time to do your Re-Do is right before you go to bed, because the time before you fall asleep is an especially potent time for repatterning your thoughts and behaviors. Your conscious mind is winding down, and your subconscious mind is opening up. Stretch out, get comfy, close your eyes, and re-do. You'll be amazed at how quickly your new, positive behaviors start occurring in your day-to-day life. That said, I recommend re-doing only one action from your day per day. Your evenings should not be about re-doing every moment of your life. Give yourself a break.

Someone Who Tried This Before You

A few years ago, my family vacationed in Central America. One day we squeezed in a scenic hike before lunch, so we didn't sit down to eat until almost three in the afternoon, and by that time I was ravenous. We ordered our food at a sleepy little hut, and it took more than an hour for it to arrive. Not only was it late, but much of our food was served without having been cooked through. It wasn't my finest hour: I turned into a protective, hungry mama bear. I marched into the kitchen and complained. I wonder, has extreme hunger ever brought out your crazy? Afterward, I realized my reaction was way out of proportion to the situation, and I apologized to everyone who'd been subjected to my rant.

I also took a few moments to imagine how I could have behaved better. I imagined myself in that situation, noticing the hunger and realizing that it's just a feeling. Starvation for the kids and me was not imminent, and we would survive. I then asked myself how I would like to have felt in that situation. I imagined feeling calm and relaxed, even though the hunger was uncomfortable. I then imagined myself in future situations feeling composed and relaxed and behaving calmly.

Sure enough, a couple months later I had an opportunity to test my work when a dinner planned for 6:15 P.M. wasn't served until 9:00. Though I was extremely hungry during those intervening hours, I managed to pass on the bread basket (I didn't want a meal based solely on simple carbs) and maintain a civilized conversation. I even managed to eat slowly and enjoy my meal once it finally arrived. My Re-Do became my reality.

The Calm Before the Storm

Once you're comfortable with the Re-Do, try another self-correcting visualization exercise. This time, combine your rethinking of past actions with plans for future behavior, called a Pre-Do. It's easy to guess what a Pre-Do is: it's simply a Re-Do for the future instead of the past. For example, if you have a birthday dinner, family event, or vacation coming up and you're concerned about overeating, you can pre-do the experiences to set yourself up for success. The key in such situations, as in the Re-Dos, is to focus on the feeling state that will allow you to make good decisions even when the unexpected happens. If you are feeling centered, balanced, and relaxed, for example, you will be much more likely to make good, healthful decisions than you would if you were stressed and anxious.

Dig In: The Pre-Do

Want to give the Pre-Do a try? Here's how it works.

1. Think of an upcoming situation you would like to go well.
2. Imagine what feeling state you would like to have during that situation. Centered? Safe? Accepted? Relaxed? Also ask yourself, "How do I want to feel *after* the dinner (work party, family reunion, etc.)?" Imagine feeling that way now.
3. Imagine yourself feeling that way in the future situation. See yourself behaving as you would like to and feeling good.
4. Really feel the good feelings of behaving in this new way.
5. Imagine a blank screen. This will signal to your mind that you have finished a complete behavior pattern. Remember: the subconscious needs to know clearly when the new behavior starts and when it finishes so it can run the behavior on automatic in real life.
6. Repeat at least three times. The more you practice in your mind, the more easily the new behaviors will take hold in your life.

Because you never know exactly what the future will bring, it's a good idea to rehearse several different scenarios from the probable to the unlikely, all based on your good-feeling state, so you will be better able to adapt to whatever happens. Again, the most important part of both the Re-Do and the Pre-Do is to cultivate a positive, feel-good state that will support your future actions, no matter how events unfold.

Both the Pre-Do and the Re-Do come in especially handy for big holiday and celebratory meals. With calorie-abundant food everywhere, and often accompanying stress caused by family members, such events can be excellent learning opportunities that allow for transformative growth. A day before a big meal such as Thanksgiving or Christmas dinner, for example, is a perfect opportunity to get your mental game plan together. Re-do your past Thanksgiving and Christmas dinners, especially if you have any negative emotional charge about past turkey-day meals. Re-do how you wish you would have felt and behaved (taken less gravy, eaten more green beans, whatever it may be). Remember to let yourself feel the good feelings associated with your reimagined outcome.

Next, pre-do how you want the day to go the next time around. Imagine enjoying every bite on your plate and positively engaging with the people you're sharing the meal with. Imagine feeling good about yourself during and after the meal. Finally, make a plan ahead of time for how you will renew should you slip up and overeat.

Overeating happens—big deal! Just have a plan in place to self-correct and get back into a positive, feel-good state after the caloric high from the pumpkin pie wears off and before the "I shouldn't have eaten all that food" guilt sets in.

Food for Thought

Before you go to a "big" meal, such as a celebratory dinner, special party, or fancy banquet, the questions to ask yourself are "How do I want to feel at the end of this evening? How do I want to feel walking out of this restaurant? Walking out of this party?" As soon as you answer those questions, you've given your subconscious mind a target to aim for.

A Little Forgiveness

As we move on to Week 4 of the Full-Filled program, I want you to begin to flirt with the idea of forgiveness. Your slip-ups provide you with rich opportunities to learn from and modify your behaviors, and they also give you an opportunity to forgive yourself for being imperfect. Forgiveness comes from truly and deeply understanding that positive intent is at the core of all your unhealthful eating habits. You want to feel good, safe, comforted, accepted, and loved. Sometimes you seek those good feelings through food, and that's okay. We've all been there! You're imperfect—welcome to the human race! Give yourself a break, and recognize and accept that wanting to feel good is a forgivable act.

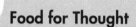

Food for Thought

Many of my clients are distraught that they've let themselves get as big as they have and wasted so much of their lives in the process. Because they are full of shame and regret, they feel completely unworthy of forgiveness. Perhaps you, too, feel that you don't deserve to be forgiven. Yet isn't that the point of true forgiveness? We are all worthy of it.

Forgiveness is an important piece of the Full-Filled program. Though forgiving yourself may be hard for you to do (beating yourself up probably comes much more easily), I encourage you to give it a try. Take a deep breath, and allow yourself to simply let go of any tension or stresses from the day. Spend the next five minutes in this mindful meditation, "A Little Forgiveness."

Mindful Meditation: A Little Forgiveness

Think about the last time you overate, discovered your clothes no longer fit, or jumped onto the scale and watched the number climb higher than it was the last time you weighed yourself. What feelings come up? Shame? Guilt? Disgust? Disappointment? Instead of beating yourself up for overeating, being overweight, or having gotten out of shape, acknowledge the positive intent of your behaviors. What is it that you've been trying so desperately to get through food? Comfort? Safety? Protection? Relief? Acceptance? Forgive yourself for wanting something good for yourself.

Now acknowledge that the situations in which you've used food to comfort yourself have been difficult ones. Before you began the Full-Filled program, the only solution you had to deal with those difficult situations and honor your positive intent was to eat. Forgive yourself for using the only tool you knew worked, for using your best coping mechanism, the best way that you could think of to renew your energy and fill you up.

Next, recognize that your mistakes and slip-ups don't identify you as a failure but instead have taught you valuable lessons. Forgive yourself for making mistakes, for being an imperfect human being who learns through mistakes just like every other human being on the planet. Could it be that your imperfections are what make you the most lovable?

Take a deep, cleansing breath in and slowly exhale any shame, guilt, regret, and disappointment from the past. Breathe in kindness, compassion, and forgiveness, and discover how wonderful and liberating it feels to let go.

You see, each time you slip up and forgive yourself for being imperfect, you acknowledge that you're worth forgiving. Funny how that works, huh? So as you continue on your weight-release journey, forgive yourself for your slip-ups, practice self-correcting, reduce your DIF, and acknowledge and appreciate your incremental steps forward. They may feel like small steps right now, yet over time they will add up to amazing breakthroughs. Just wait!

Progress Report

Over the next seven days, be sure to:

1. **Practice self-correcting *after* an overeating episode.** Self-correction is what you do to return to a feel-good, balanced state after you've been thrown off course. When you correct your course after you have strayed only slightly, you will feel better about yourself and avoid a future binge.

2. **Make a list of Level One self-correction techniques in your Full-Filled Weight-Release Journal.** These self-correcting tools are fairly quick and easy things that you can do on your own every day to rebalance yourself energetically, emotionally, spiritually, and physically in order to get back on track to feeling good. They include working out, meditating, getting a good night's rest, hydrating, eating a protein-rich breakfast, or simply running an inner dialogue that's positive, kind, and accepting. The key to these activities is that they leave you feeling renewed and better about yourself and your body than when you started.

3. **Make a list of Level Two self-correction techniques in your Full-Filled Weight-Release Journal.** When you need a boost beyond Level One techniques to rebalance and renew your energy and put you back into a feel-good state after overeating, reach out to someone else for additional support. Make a list of people who can help you get back on track. Also list social situations that will help you feel inspired and encouraged by those around you.

4. **Make a list of Level Three self-correction techniques in your Full-Filled Weight-Release Journal.** Prepare yourself should you need

the help of a professional to bring you back to your center. Identify a trained professional (traditional doctor, hypnotherapist, life coach, counselor, therapist, bodyworker, or spiritual adviser) whose help you will seek in the event that you need Level Three support. If you don't have someone in mind already, note the specific steps you will take to find someone.

5. **Track the duration, intensity, and frequency of your overeating in your weight-release journal.** One way to really notice if you are creating a slimming trend in your life is by becoming aware of how long, how much, and how often you overeat. In your weight-release journal, document the duration, intensity, and frequency of your most recent overeating episodes. After you've become aware of your current patterns, set one reasonable goal for reducing your DIF this week.

6. **Practice the Re-Do after an overeating episode.** By re-doing your past slip-up in your mind, you start the process of replacing your previous behavior pattern with a new desired one. Remember, when you re-do, really focus on feeling good as you behave in a positive way. Practice the Re-Do at least once this week right before you go to sleep. Take note of your experience in your Full-Filled Weight-Release Journal.

7. **Practice the Pre-Do.** Once you're comfortable with the Re-Do, try the Pre-Do, which is simply a Re-Do for the future instead of for the past. This time, combine your rethinking of past actions with plans for future behavior. Practice the Pre-Do at least once this week. Note your experience in your Full-Filled Weight-Release Journal.

8. **Forgive yourself for your mistakes.** Forgiveness comes from truly and deeply understanding that positive intent is at the core of all your unhealthy eating habits.

What Are You Really Hungry For?

As you continue on your weight-release journey, you will occasionally overeat, then self-correct and modify your eating habits, which will get you closer and closer to the body and life you so passionately desire. You will continue to discover that your slip-ups are opportunities to self-correct. On top of that, you're about to learn that your slip-ups are like flashing red arrows pointing you directly to the root of your weight struggle.

You see, each trip to the cookie jar is a clear signal that a part of you is asking for deep healing. Underneath the surface, some unresolved discontent or pain continues to drive you towards the temporary satisfaction—or distraction—of food.

This week, you will work to release and heal this pain so you're no longer triggered to overeat. When you break this pain-triggered cycle, food simply becomes nourishment. Pain, an inevitable part of life, simply becomes short-lived pain.

If the prospect excites you, it should. This week is all about big-time transformation that will benefit your waistline and every other area of your life.

In Week 4 of the Full-Filled program, you will learn to:
- Identify your trigger situations and trigger foods
- Name the limiting beliefs holding you back

- Use the EFT to transform your limiting beliefs into empowering beliefs
- Forgive and accept yourself as you are today

As you begin Week 4 of the Full-Filled program, **set your intention to gently and compassionately identify and release what's been holding you back from having the body, life, and relationship with food that you dream of**. Take a deep, cleansing breath and become present with your intention. It's in the present that change is possible.

Once your intention is firmly rooted in your mind and before you dive into this week of the program, I want to pause for a moment to acknowledge that it can feel a bit overwhelming to dig into pain that you weren't aware of or that you've been consciously trying to avoid much of your life. Let's reflect on this.

You've already done a lot of deep, reflective work over the past few weeks. And I bet you've come further in this program than you even realize. That's because when real, deep, and lasting change happens, it's often subtle, and therefore it's very easy to forget what life was like before the shift. That's because of the success amnesia that kicks in (I introduced this concept in Week 1). This is when a habit or a thought you had disappears so thoroughly that you forget you ever had it. It's very possible that success amnesia has already happened to you.

A client named Roger who enrolled in a group I ran came up at the end of the program and thanked me for helping him lose 25 pounds. I said to him, "Wow. That's fantastic. What changed?"

He thought about it for a minute and said, "I'm not really sure. Nothing's changed, except . . . I don't eat potato chips anymore."

I said, "How is it that you stopped eating them?"

"I can't really say," he said. "I'm just not buying them."

I reminded him that he'd told the group early on that for twenty-five years, he'd had a habit of overeating potato chips. No matter how hard he tried, he couldn't resist eating them.

"And now you're not buying them?" I asked. "When did you stop?"

"Good question," he answered. "I'd have to think about it."

"Was it after you did the work in this program to release that specific compulsion?" I asked.

"I guess it was," he said. "But that didn't help."

"Oh?" I replied. "How do you know it didn't work?"

"Because I could tell everyone else in the program was doing the exercise better than me."

"So you had a compulsion to eat potato chips for twenty-five years, and you lost that compulsion around the time you did an exercise in this class to lose the compulsion." I smiled. "And do you think that's pure coincidence?"

"Wait a minute—do you think that's why I stopped eating them?"

Roger was completely unaware that the deep work he had done in the program had worked so thoroughly that his desire to buy potato chips—the food he had loved most—had totally disappeared.

Take a few moments now to acknowledge the progress you've already made so far in your weight-release journey. Take a look back at your answers to the Dig In exercises from Weeks 1, 2, and 3. Notice how far you've already come, not just for the fun of it but because by appreciating and noticing your progress, you nurture the positive seeds of change that you planted weeks ago and help them take deeper root.

Understanding Triggers

I once had a client who, when I asked her what triggered her to overeat, replied, "Breathing." When she thought about it a bit more, she narrowed it down to "being awake." It may seem as though your overeating is so out of control and random that anything and everything triggers you to empty the refrigerator, but in reality, I think you'll discover exactly what my client did: there are really only a few types of trigger situations that set you off and cause you to overdo it. It's just that they happen over and over again.

For example, maybe you're someone who can't stop from tearing into the chips when you're home alone at night. Or maybe you're driven to load up on free munchies when you're in social settings, such as work parties or happy hour with friends. Perhaps you clean off your kids' plates after they leave the dinner table. Or maybe you raid the vending machine when you're planning for a client meeting or studying for an exam.

Once you start paying attention to these patterns, you will realize that there are only a few specific situations in your life in which you feel triggered to overeat. Take a look back at your answers to the Dig In exercise from Week 1 when I asked you to catalog the specific behaviors you wanted to change, and I bet they'll reveal some of your triggers.

Eating is a way to escape or suppress bad feelings and to feel good ones instead, even if you aren't consciously aware of it in the moment—and most people aren't. So identifying your triggers is the most direct and effective way to get to the root of any unhealed pain that's holding you back. By identifying your triggers, you can curb a lot of your mouth-stuffing moments, so start the process by asking yourself, "What gets me eating? What specific situations set me off on an all-out eating rampage?"

At the height of my binge eating, my top trigger situation was being home alone at night. I was a hard-core sugar junkie then, and I'd turn the kitchen upside down looking for anything sweet. Cake, cookies, candy, ice cream—I just couldn't get enough. In fact, in college I went on an all-sugar diet. My lunch of choice was an ice-cream cone with a side of chocolate-covered peanuts (for the protein). By three o'clock, I'd have a terrible blood sugar crash, which I quickly fixed with a candy bar. Take it from me, this nutritional approach is not a good one. The extreme highs and lows of all-sugar-all-the-time turn you into a moody mess and take a toll on your health.

In the Dig In exercise below, you will begin developing a deeper awareness of your triggers. Take out a pen or pencil, and in the table below or in your Full-Filled Weight-Release Journal, list your trigger situations in order of frequency. In other words, list first the situation that comes up the most frequently and that, 90 percent of the time, causes you to head face-first into the food.

Dig In: What Are Your Triggers?

List your trigger situations in order of frequency. In other words, list first the trigger whose release would make the biggest positive difference in your life. For example, "If I could stop snacking late at night, I would eat so much less (plus I'd sleep better)." *Trigger situation: late-night eating.*

Rank   Trigger Situation

———— ————————————————————————————

———— ————————————————————————————

———— ————————————————————————————

———— ————————————————————————————

———— ————————————————————————————

You may also have certain trigger foods that set you off again and again. These are the foods that, no matter how hard you try, you just can't seem to eat in moderation. In fact, eating just one bite of these provoking foods (e.g., cookies, potato chips) triggers you to eat ten to twenty more. Take a moment now to list your worst trigger foods—changing your compulsion to eat these to a take-it-or-leave-it attitude would make the biggest positive difference in your life. For example, "If I could resist the midmorning latte and muffin run, I'd consume a lot fewer calories." *Trigger food: muffins at the coffee bar.*

Rank	Trigger Foods
____	_____
____	_____
____	_____
____	_____
____	_____

After you've completed your trigger lists, sit with this information for a few minutes. What do you think it is about these particular situations or foods that triggers you to overeat? Do you have any idea? To spark further insight, take a look at what you've written down and notice what, if any, feelings or memories come up for you when you think about being triggered to eat in each of these situations. Keep those thoughts at the front of your mind as I walk you through the next several steps.

To get to the root of why certain situations trigger you to overeat, you will dig in just as you did in Week 2 when you learned how to uncover the bad feelings that drive you to overeat and name the good feelings (i.e., positive intent) that you'd like to experience instead.

 Food for Thought

Remember, there is no such thing as "blowing it" in the Full-Filled program. Every experience you have, every time you overeat or binge, supports your success. Overeating episodes, full-on binges, and even minor overeating are pointers that make your work easier. They point to a trigger situation that is up for releasing. They tell you what to heal next.

I also want you to revisit from Week 2 the example of indulging in an afternoon candy bar. To uncover why this situation triggers overeating, you mentally rewound to the moment right before you headed to the vending machine. You realized that you were feeling exhausted and run down and wanted the lift that chocolate would temporarily provide. Upon further inspection, you discovered that underneath your feelings of exhaustion were the thoughts "I've been working like a dog, and there's still more to be done. I'm afraid I won't get it all done in time." After digging a little deeper, you uncovered a more acute fear: "If I can't get it all done, that will mean I'm a failure, and I'll get fired and end up a bag lady on the street."

In that scenario you were the Overachieving Multitasker, and long hours in the office triggered you to overeat because the work environment provoked feelings of insecurity and unworthiness in you. *Trigger situation: long hours at the office, because they tend to bring up feelings of insecurity and unworthiness.*

Dig In: The Trigger Beneath the Trigger

Take a moment now to dig into the first trigger situation on your list. Ask yourself, "What feelings come up in this specific situation that trigger me to overeat?" Dig deep. Imagine that you are in the situation. Rewind to the moment right before you felt the urge to eat and play your thoughts back in s-l-o-w motion. (You can also do this exercise with your weight-release buddy, asking her to help you re-create the situation in your mind. Sometimes having a friend guide you can produce insights that you wouldn't get on your own.)

Once you've stepped back to the moment right before you felt the urge to eat, notice your thoughts. What are you feeling? If feelings of dissatisfaction have risen to the surface, you're right on track.

More often than not, you will experience a moment of acute pain or discomfort that hasn't been healed—that is what triggers you to overeat. Identify the negative feeling or feelings that set you off, and write them down in your weight-release journal. Then set this exercise aside. We're going to build on it in a minute.

Again, let's revisit that office bingeing scenario from Week 2. For the Overachieving Multitasker, her positive intent for eating is to get a break from all her relentless doing while giving herself extra energy to do even more. Still, true satisfaction evades her because she thinks she can never do enough or do well enough to earn a lasting sense of self-worth—and ultimately that's what she wants most.

Last week, you began honoring the positive intent of your overeating and excess weight with daily self-care and self-correction tools instead of with food. No doubt you've noticed how much better having a good night's rest, exercising, or talking with a trusted friend feels than cleaning your plate and going back for more. Yet there are likely to be certain situations that still trigger you to overeat almost automatically. And no, it's not just because you love food! If it were, you would honor the food you eat by savoring every bite and eating when you most enjoy it—when you have a good appetite. We'll talk more about this in Week 5. For now, suffice it to say that underneath your trigger is something that you're probably unaware of. Can you guess what it is?

I'll give you a hint. Okay, I'll give you a big hint: *fear*. Remember from Week 2 that underneath the bad feelings that often drive or trigger you to overeat are universal fears. The Overachieving Multitasker, for example, fears that she's not good enough.

Whatever your particular trigger situation—being home alone at night, mingling at social gatherings, sitting down to family dinner, or passing through the office break room—it triggers a fear that you haven't yet healed. And that fear—that you're unworthy, underappreciated, unsafe, or imperfect—is driving you to overeat. Although you've been working with some of my favorite self-care and self-correction tools to help you feel that you *are* worthy, appreciated, safe, and good enough without reaching for the munchies, some amount of fear is still alive and kicking, and it's as if every time you overeat, your deepest fear is making the point: *Release me! I'm still here!*

The wonderful news is that the simple tools that you are about to learn will allow you to completely release even your biggest fears and, with them, your triggers. How great is that? Imagine how amazing it will be to forget to overeat in your old trigger situations. Imagine going to a party or an event and barely noticing the buffet table as you focus instead on the people you enjoy most. Imagine feeling relaxed and peaceful after dinner as you settle into your favorite wind-down activity, be it reading, journaling, watching TV, or talking to a friend on the phone. Imagine losing your desire to overeat and in exchange gaining an overall sense of satisfaction that fills you up like nothing else. Can you imagine that for yourself? The way to get there is not by depriving and controlling your behaviors but by addressing the thoughts and feelings that trigger you to overeat. And when you approach weight loss in this deep and profound way, not only will you drop the pounds, you'll also become more fully present in your life. That's the hidden bonus of the Full-Filled program. I want you to think about that bonus as you dig into the next phase of the program.

 Food for Thought

The next time that you have an eating episode that makes you feel a little bit bad, or maybe even very bad, and you feel that you've really blown it, say "thank you" to that episode. A client who had overdone it on an enormous burrito felt both physically awful and guilty afterward. Yet we were able to use that episode to point to a deep trigger for her: her feelings of abandonment from being neglected and mistreated as a child. In the end she said, "Thank you, big burrito!" The big burrito became her teacher, because a slip is a big pointer. It's a big opportunity to resolve a trigger situation that's still holding you back.

Changing Self-Limiting Beliefs

Like everything else you've done so far in this program, releasing your fears is a process, and I will walk you through it step by step. The first step to releasing your fears is to get underneath them and identify what's causing them. In other words, you need to figure out where the heck they're coming from.

To answer this question, let's look back at one of the most pervasive personality types introduced in Week 2: the Giver. She is the selfless mother, the devoted daughter, and the loyal friend who puts everyone else's needs before her own. She eats in an attempt to replenish her energy because her constant giving leaves her emotionally, spiritually, and physically drained. She could give a little less and take care of herself more, but she fears she's not deserving of the same love and care she bestows on others. Where do you think this fear comes from? Any ideas? It comes from the limiting belief that she's unworthy, and it's that belief that holds her back from a slim, healthful, and fulfilling life.

A belief is something you consider to be true whether or not you have conclusive evidence—just like having spiritual faith. Though there is no proof that God exists, believers just "know" in their guts and hearts that God is real. When you have a belief that holds you back, it's called a limiting belief because you believe it to be true even though it limits your life experience in some way. A self-limiting belief can easily shortchange your professional success, your physical and emotional health, and your overall sense of happiness and well-being.

Take, for example, the story of Robert Dilts, one of the founders of NLP (neurolinguistic programming) and a coauthor of *Beliefs: Pathways to Health & Well-Being*. In the book, Dilts wrote that his mother had a recurrence of breast cancer. She was very sick and believed wholeheartedly that she would die. "Cancer causes death" was her belief. Dilts decided to see if belief change would help her improve her health in any way. He began by asking his mother, "Does cancer *always* cause death?" After thinking about it, she said, "No, it does not." He spent four days questioning her beliefs and fears about cancer and, more important, her beliefs about herself and her own self-worth. After four days of intensive work, Dilts was able to help his mother release a whole bag of limiting beliefs she'd been carrying around. Not long after that, her cancer went into full remission. True story.

Food for Thought

By following the Full-Filled program, you will undermine and eventually completely release the old mind-set that's been keeping you away from the body and life of your dreams. The tools outlined in the pages ahead will work for you by undermining the specific mentality, the specific mind-set, of the weight struggle. There's a whole system of thinking and beliefs in our society that creates the weight struggle. But you can change those beliefs and transform your struggle into peace, enjoyment, and a fulfilling life.

Limiting beliefs have a very sneaky way of validating themselves. If, for example, you believe you're going to die of cancer, the chances are good that you will. Similarly, if you believe you're not good enough, worthy, or lovable, then guess what? You will, more than likely, become the selfless Giver who gives and never receives. Likewise, if you hold a strong negative image of yourself that differs from what the people around you see, such as regarding yourself as "huge" when in reality you're a slim size eight, you will unconsciously find or create evidence to support your conviction. The mind becomes confused by contradictory thoughts, so in an effort to resolve the discrepancy between your belief system and reality, your subconscious mind will act like a magnet, attracting experiences or circumstances to your life that reinforce what you passionately believe. In other words, your persistent fat thoughts will attract a fat body.

I've lost count of the number of clients who have long seen themselves as fat. I used to see myself that way, too. A client who came to me with 150 pounds to release had always been told she was fat. She had been sent to fat camps as a child and spent a lifetime feeling bad about how she looked. This "fat thinking" significantly influenced her behaviors and life experiences. Yet when she and I looked back at pictures of her as a child, she realized how slim and healthy she'd actually been. She hadn't been fat at all, but because she had been told she was fat, she had believed she was, and her belief that she was overweight had become a self-fulfilling prophecy.

Food for Thought

The belief that we can change and that healing is possible is what inside-out weight loss is all about. It's about the magical transformation that happens when we change what we believe—when we realize that we can change, that it is possible.

While self-limiting beliefs determine a great deal of our life experiences, we are typically unaware of them and how they influence some of our most automatic behaviors, such as eating. Because most of our beliefs were created when we were children, they have long ago slipped into our subconscious minds. Your work throughout this next section will be to bring your limiting beliefs to conscious awareness so you can change them into empowering beliefs that will attract the body and life you truly want and deserve.

Someone Who Tried This Before You

Christi, a beautiful woman in her twenties with clear blue eyes and a captivating smile, came to me to lose 30 pounds.

As she began to release the weight, she found herself struggling with her eating again, so we dived deeper into the upside of being overweight. When I asked her to imagine being exactly as she wanted to be, she began to feel uneasy. The more she thought about it, the more she realized that she had objections to releasing weight—if she were slim, she would have no more excuses for not being as successful as she felt she should be. She would have to face the reality of her perceived failures. Her excess weight helped her avoid the pain of facing her own faults.

It turned out that the high standards Christi held herself to were actually her father's standards, which she had never been able to meet. Christi believed that her father never thought she was good enough, and she struggled with her deep desire to gain love and acceptance from him. To that end, she pushed herself to unrealistic standards while becoming very good at not measuring up to them, just as her father expected. Christi was playing out her father's limiting beliefs about her.

When Christi realized that the part of her that was overeating really just wanted love and acceptance, she broke down in my office, crying in relief. With my guidance, she was able to release her fear of failure and begin the process of accepting and loving her deepest self. Not long after that, her eating struggles began to disappear.

To bring your limiting beliefs to conscious awareness, go back to the Dig In exercise "The Trigger Beneath the Trigger" on page 120 and pick up where you left off. You identified the negative feelings that automatically trigger you to overeat, and I trust that you wrote them down in your Full-Filled Weight-Release Journal. If not, write them down now so you can build on that awareness in the next Dig In exercise.

Dig In: What Are Your Limiting Beliefs?

As you contemplate the negative feelings that trigger you to go hog wild at a buffet table or fast-food restaurant, I want you to allow yourself to open up to the fear associated with those feelings. I know, there are other activities that sound like a lot more fun, but trust me; there will be a payoff for the next few uncomfortable moments. Ask yourself, "What is my biggest fear? What's my worst-case scenario? That my boss will figure out I'm not up to snuff? That I can't succeed in my relationships because I'm not really lovable?" Slowly breathe in and out and sit with the painful feelings associated with your fear. As you continue to breathe, ask yourself, "Where does this fear come from? What core limiting beliefs do I have that support this fear?" You may get the answer in a flash, or it may take some reflection. If you're not accustomed to slowing down your thought process so much, be patient with yourself. What you don't become aware of now will become clear over time.

If you're not sure you're getting the "right" insights or your limiting beliefs feel too embarrassing or shameful to write down, take a minute to read over some of the most common limiting beliefs that clients have shared with me over the years:

I am not worthy or deserving of care or love.

I am inadequate—not smart enough, pretty enough, rich enough, and so on.

I am a fraud on every level—at work, in friendships, and in family relationships.

I am a failure and a disappointment.

I am misunderstood and underappreciated.

I will never fit in.

I will always be lonely and empty.

I must always protect myself because the world is a dangerous place.

If I really love someone, I will get hurt.

If I show the true me, I will be rejected.

Do any of these limiting beliefs resonate with you? I wouldn't be surprised if they did. They are some of our most universal fears. How do you think these limiting beliefs play into your body image and your ability to drop weight and keep it off?

If you believe that you're not deserving of love and happiness, you may also believe that you don't deserve to be slim and healthy for a lifetime.

If you believe you must always protect yourself, you likely believe it's unsafe to be thin.

If you believe you're inadequate, you might also believe that you're incapable of making healthful choices and controlling yourself around food.

If you believe you'll never fit in, you probably believe you'll never be able to change or become "thin enough."

And if you believe you're a disappointment, you may believe that successfully losing weight eventually leads to regaining it and to failure.

I had a client who absolutely believed the last one. Every time he lost weight, he'd celebrate by taking himself out to an Italian meal, where he'd load up on lasagna and garlic bread. He had a pattern of "success sabotage." His limiting belief that success only led to failure was so firmly rooted in his subconscious mind that every time he dropped a few pounds, he would unconsciously find a way to support his limiting belief—by eating his way back up the scale!

Food for Thought

As you uncover your limiting beliefs, be patient with yourself; sometimes beliefs reveal themselves all at once, and sometimes they reveal themselves over time. Tune in to them, and be excited when you discover one. Whenever I stumble upon a limiting belief that's held me back in some way, I think, "Wow, great. Now I can change it." And off I go.

Can you see that limiting beliefs such as the ones above hold you back from having the life and body of your dreams? I wonder if you can also identify what they all have in common. They suggest a lack of personal power and efficacy. They're actually beliefs about helplessness, hopelessness, and worthlessness. These three types of limiting beliefs are the most pervasive in our diet and body image–obsessed culture. Clients readily tell me:

I can't lose weight because I've never lost it before.

If I lose weight, I'll gain it back.

I can't lose weight because my family is overweight.

Weight loss is impossibly hard. I'll never have the body I truly desire.

I don't deserve to be happy.

These are all code phrases for "I feel worthless. I don't believe I deserve to change" or "I feel helpless. I don't believe I can change" or "I feel hopeless. I don't believe that change is possible." Amy, a client of mine, told me, "Well, you know, I'm just a big girl. I've always been big. My parents were big, and I've always been chubby. It's hard for me to believe that I could ever be anything different." That limiting belief was holding Amy back. She didn't believe that she could ever be anything different, and if she didn't believe she could be slim and healthy, it was going to be very difficult for her to ever change. I wonder, do you think you have the power to change? Do you think it's possible to change?

The answer is yes! Nod your head affirmatively up and down. Change is possible. It happened for me. It's happened for countless others who have followed this program, and I'll show you exactly how it can now happen for you.

Dig In: Limiting Beliefs About Weight and Weight Release

To help you uncover how your limiting beliefs play into your eating habits, weight, and body image, try this free-form journaling exercise. Complete the following sentences in your Full-Filled Weight-Release Journal.

1. Losing weight is . . .

2. I'm overweight because . . .

Write down everything that comes to mind. Being truthful with yourself will provide you with the biggest insights. Once you've completed the exercise, see if you can pull out your limiting beliefs. For example, "Losing weight is hard work." "Losing weight is painful." "Losing weight is scary."

"I'm overweight because it's in my genes. I have big bones and a slow metabolism." "I'm overweight because I'm lazy." "I'm overweight because I'm a failure at everything."

After free-form journaling for a while, don't be surprised if you identify one of the big three limiting beliefs: hopelessness, helplessness, or worthlessness. For example, "I'm overweight because I don't deserve to be slim" is fueled by a belief in worthlessness. "Losing weight means I have to be perfect" has roots in helplessness. "I'm overweight because that's how I've always been" is a belief about hopelessness.

Change Your Limiting Beliefs

Because your beliefs, to a great extent, create your reality, you can change much of your life by simply changing your beliefs. And since you are the creator of the limiting beliefs you hold now, you have the power to create new, empowering beliefs to replace them. When you transform your limiting beliefs about helplessness, hopelessness, and worthlessness into empowering beliefs, the benefits typically extend far beyond skipping the double fries and watching your waistline shrink. When you change from a limiting belief such as "I'm not worthy or deserving of happiness" to believing you can create your life as you want it and are worthy of it to boot, your work life, home life, relationships, and friendships—all aspects of your life—benefit from the change. That is why changing beliefs is so powerful, transformative, and exciting! I wonder, how many positive changes in your life will result as you transform your limiting beliefs into empowering beliefs?

Someone Who Tried This Before You

A client of mine named Sam had a breakthrough moment one day when he was telling a coworker how sore his neck was. His coworker said that he was surprised that Sam was in pain because he never seemed to be in pain. That got Sam thinking about pain and about the emotional pain we carry around that is not often visible to people around us. At that moment, Sam realized the "gift" his weight had been trying to give him for years. He came to understand that his weight had been serving to protect him from emotional pain.

Sam explained to me that he'd always been afraid to let others see the "real" him. "I've always been very empathetic, but when it comes to my own feelings and deep connections, I've always shielded that part of me with anger and sarcasm . . . and now I'm coming to understand that I've used my excess weight to shield me as well."

He had been a heavy child. "Because I was heavy, I always had something obvious for people to pick on me about. In a way, my weight kept people distracted and away from other areas in my life that might actually be more sensitive for me," such as relationships.

As an adult, Sam was using his weight to protect himself from the emotional pain that can often accompany romantic entanglements. "I believe my fear of the intense emotional pain that can come with failed relationships has held me back."

After identifying his objections to releasing weight and the gift that his weight had been giving him all these years (protection and procrastination), he dug deeper to uncover the fears and limiting beliefs supporting his weight struggle.

Sam discovered that he held a key limiting belief. He didn't believe he was strong enough to deal emotionally with the possibility of the severe pain that comes from a failed relationship. "The mere idea of a relationship—allowing someone to get that close—scares me, and what would happen if it blew up? The thought almost brings me to tears and makes me want to hide. It makes me not even want to consider losing weight and becoming attractive to the opposite sex, because it then places me much closer to that [potential] situation."

I commended Sam for doing such deep, introspective work and told him that the key to releasing his limiting belief about helplessness was to begin questioning it. By introducing doubt to your limiting beliefs, you begin to release the stranglehold they have on you.

Beliefs have a magnetic quality: they attract evidence that supports them, which makes you miss or dismiss evidence to the contrary. The way to change limiting beliefs, then, is by questioning them. Much as how Robert Dilts questioned his mother's belief that cancer causes death, you will question your limiting beliefs to find they are much more doubtful than you thought.

Dig In: Question Your Old Beliefs

Choose one of your limiting beliefs from the list you created earlier. Pick the one with the biggest emotional charge or the one whose release would make the biggest positive difference in your life.

Start to question it. Your goal is not to outright disprove the belief but to open it up to questioning and doubt. Imagine that you are an innocent child and are really trying to understand this belief and question every aspect of it. Write anything that comes to mind in your weight-release journal. For example, if your old belief is "I'm not good enough," what happens when you question this belief?

Ask yourself, "How do I know I'm not good enough? Who decides who's good enough? How would I know if I were good enough? Do I know anyone who *is* good enough? Does being good enough make people more lovable?"

After you question and introduce doubt to your old belief, start looking for and writing down evidence about why it might not be true, why it might be completely false. Look for instances that disprove it. These are called counterexamples. For example, if you believe it's not possible for you to release weight and stay slim, ask, "Is it possible for anyone?" Then consider, "Well, Renée did it, and lots of people who follow this program have done it, so it must be possible. If it was possible for them, why wouldn't it be possible for me? Is there something about me that makes it impossible for me to lose weight when it's possible for others?" You answer, "No, I'm no different from anyone else. If it's possible for them, it must be possible for me, too."

Many people who struggle with their weight believe they cannot change because they haven't succeeded before. I get that, but consider this: maybe it's simply that you didn't have the right tools before.

Imagine standing at a doorway blocked by thick wooden boards that are screwed into the door frame. You desperately want to pass through, but the boards make it impossible. The only tool you have on hand to remove them is a hammer. You bang and bang and bang on the boards, exhausting yourself, tears of frustration rolling down your face because you really, really want to pass through. Alas, the hammer is the wrong tool for this job. After cursing yourself and cursing the ineffectiveness of the hammer, someone walks up and hands you a screwdriver. You unscrew the screws, and each board comes off quickly and easily, until they are all removed and you pass through with ease. With the right tools, a job that used to be impossible or extremely difficult becomes easy. That's what I'm giving you here.

Once you start to question your limiting beliefs, I think you'll find it becomes harder and harder to believe them, and that's because they often don't make much rational sense. Your growing doubt, in combination with questioning their validity, will eventually break them down, making plenty of room for new, empowering beliefs that will enhance your life. How great is that?

Food for Thought

Often the limiting beliefs that hold the most power over us, when brought out into the light of day, sound downright ridiculous. The enjoyable thing about identifying a limiting belief with your weight-release buddy is that together you can laugh at them. And laughter is one of the most effective belief busters I know of.

Making the Switch to Empowering Beliefs

Empowering beliefs are the opposite of limiting beliefs. For example, the opposite of "I will never fit in" is the empowering belief "I am lovable exactly as I am." When crafting new, empowering beliefs, be sure to state them in the positive. For example, "My essence is good" is much more powerful than "I'm not a bad person." Say each version to yourself, and notice how each one makes you feel. Also, make sure they are all in the present tense. If you create an empowering belief for the future, it will remain in the future, always just ahead of where you are. For example, if your limiting belief is that it's hard work to lose weight, your new, empowering belief could be "It's easy and natural to be a healthy, slim weight." If your old belief is that it's not possible to make lasting change, a new, empowering belief might be "I am always on a journey of learning, growing, and improving." Finally, make sure that your new belief is believable (if it's not, your rational mind will dismiss it). When changing your old beliefs into empowering beliefs, start with something that is simple and unarguable and that makes you feel good when you say it. Here are a few examples to get you going:

I am loved.

I am safe.

I feel good about myself.

I am worthy of radiant health.

I love feeling great in my body.

I love making the most healthful choices.

I deserve to take great care of me.

I deeply love and accept myself.

My body craves health and balance.

My best body is easily creating itself.

Dig In: Create Empowering Beliefs

Create a new, empowering belief by first writing down your old belief on the left side of a page in your weight-release journal and then writing the opposite of that belief on the right side of the page. Be sure to state your empowering belief positively and in the present. For example, you can replace your old belief "I'm a fraud. Others will soon find out who I really am" with any of the following empowering beliefs: "I am perfectly imperfect, like all human beings." "My imperfections make me lovable." "I am most loved when I am my authentic self." Refine your empowering belief until it feels just right.

After you've crafted the new, empowering belief that you want for yourself, try it on for size by using it as an affirmation, a simple positive statement that you repeat to yourself. The key to a good affirmation is to create one that makes you feel really good when you say it. Repeat your new, empowering belief to yourself over and over again to see how you like it. Repeat it while standing in line, while driving, while doing the dishes or the laundry or whatever it is that you do. Again, pay particular attention to how this new belief makes you feel. This is very important. I want you to notice how it feels in your body and then let the wording of your new belief evolve, if appropriate. You might start off with a statement such as "I am safe and healthy" and change it to "I *feel* safe and healthy" because, perhaps by tweaking the statement from "I am" to "I feel," you get a deeper positive hit. Play around with your new, empowering beliefs until they fit you just right.

Food for Thought

If you have a belief such as "I'm not worth it," imagine changing that belief and what it will feel like on a truly deep level to know that you are worth treating wonderfully. The limiting beliefs that have been causing you to overeat have likely been limiting you in other ways, too, so when you change them, you get benefits that ripple throughout many different areas of your life. I wonder, what indirect benefits will you experience from the work you're doing in this program? I wonder, what will you notice first?

The Emotional Freedom Technique

After you begin the work of transforming your old, limiting beliefs into empowering beliefs, it's important to release the emotional hold that your old beliefs have on you. To release the negative feelings and thoughts associated with your limiting beliefs, you will use the Emotional Freedom Technique. EFT is a powerful tool for releasing negative thoughts, fears, frustrations, and limiting beliefs and replacing them with positive thoughts. "One tool that does all that?" you ask. Does it sound too good to be true? I bet it does, but remember, when you have the right tools, what seemed impossible before becomes not just possible but even easy. The Emotional Freedom Technique works quite quickly and effectively, and you can do it almost anytime, anywhere, in just a few minutes. It may seem complex when you first learn it, but you will soon be able to do it easily after just a few rounds of practice because the basic format stays the same.

What Is the Emotional Freedom Technique?

I have to admit that when I first learned that the Emotional Freedom Technique involved tapping, humming, and singing nursery rhymes, I said, "This is way too weird for me." Honest to goodness, that's what I said. "There is no way I'm teaching this to my clients. It's too out there!" What happened? Now I'm a huge fan of the Emotional Freedom Technique, and that's because I had an amazing personal breakthrough with this tool when I learned a simplified version of it from my dear friend the talented healer Gina Orlando, who is a skilled, compassionate hypnotherapist and wellness coach in the Chicago area. As you may have figured out by now, I love simple, fast, and effective tools, and that's exactly what the Emotional Freedom Technique is. In fact, I haven't come across a better technique for do-it-yourself emotional clearing work. What I used to think would take years of therapy to release can typically be released with a few rounds of the Emotional Freedom Technique.

My favorite metaphor for describing how the Emotional Freedom Technique works is a hot, steamy shower stall, one where the hot water's been going for a really long time and the steam is so thick you could cut it with a knife. When you open the door of the shower stall, all of the steam escapes, allowing fresh air to come rushing in. That's kind of how the Emotional Freedom Technique works. Over the years, your fears, limiting beliefs, and negative thoughts and feelings have built up inside you, clouding your spiritual, mental, and emotional energy. The Emotional Freedom Technique releases this fog of negative energy so the positive can filter back in.

The Emotional Freedom Technique uses the same energy meridians that have been used for thousands of years in acupuncture and Chinese medicine. These meridians are also used in practices such as tai chi and qigong and all sorts of other Asian traditions. Unlike acupuncture, however, in which needles are used on specific points on these meridian lines, with the Emotional Freedom Technique you will actually tap on the meridian points of your body with your fingers as you bring up painful emotions and speak them aloud. Though it's not yet fully understood how the Emotional Freedom Technique works, it is thought that the coordination of tapping with talking and feeling, while simultaneously stimulating the meridian points of the body, breaks apart the mental structure of your old, limiting patterns and beliefs. Once the structures have broken apart, the positive suggestion that is included in each Emotional Freedom Technique sequence readily settles into the newly available space in your subconscious mind.

The Emotional Freedom Technique, Step by Step

You can use the Emotional Freedom Technique for releasing negative thoughts, fears, frustrations, and even cravings, but you will use it at this point in the Full-Filled program to release your limiting beliefs. Don't worry if this seems a bit weird to you at first. Reserve judgment until you have your own personal breakthrough.

1. RATE YOUR FEAR ON A SCALE OF 1 TO 10.
What is your limiting belief? Bring up the painful feeling or fear associated with this belief. I recommend that you exaggerate your

feelings in your mind, because the more intensely you feel a negative charge while tapping, the more thoroughly you'll release it. I've had clients say, "I don't want to be feeling all this negative stuff. It's scary to me." I recognize that the deep work I'm asking you to do here could be a bit uncomfortable and unnerving, yet you must go to the root of your negative emotions because it's only there that you can open up that steamy shower stall and allow fresh, new air in. (Plus, I think you'll find this process quite liberating and even fun!) Imagine the weight off your shoulders, and a bunch of other places, too, as you release old beliefs and fears that have been monopolizing your energy for years. How great will that feel?

Once you've brought up the painful feeling associated with your belief, rate the strength of the negative charge on a scale of 1 to 10, with 10 being the highest and most intense. This is an important step so you can appreciate your progress (and avoid success amnesia). In fact, I encourage you to jot down your limiting belief and its intensity in your Full-Filled Weight-Release Journal before you proceed. After you've done a few rounds of the EFT, check back in and reevaluate the intensity and charge of your belief. Chances are, the intensity will have decreased. That's progress!

2. CREATE AN INTENTION STATEMENT IN THE FOLLOWING FORMAT.

Even though [limiting belief], I still deeply and completely love and accept myself.

The first part of your intention statement is the negatively charged feeling that you want to release. The second part is a positively charged affirmation. Here are some examples:

Even though I feel out of control around food, I still deeply and completely love and accept myself.

Even though I feel like a failure, I still deeply and completely love and accept myself.

Even though weight loss feels impossible, I still deeply and completely love and accept myself.

Even though losing weight feels unsafe, I still deeply and completely love and accept myself.

Even though I feel unworthy, I still deeply and completely love and accept myself.

You will notice that the positively charged affirmation is the same in each of the examples. It happens to be my personal favorite and is a great one to start with because unconditional self-acceptance and love are key components of the Full-Filled program, as you will discover before finishing this week of the program. That said, you could craft your own affirmation to complete your intention statement. Perhaps you'd like to use one of your new, empowering beliefs. Just make sure it's stated in the positive and the present. Here are a few alternative suggestions:

Even though I feel out of control around food, I choose to forgive myself and feel good about myself.

Even though losing weight feels unsafe, all is well and all will be well.

Even though I don't think I deserve to be happy, I choose to release the root causes of this belief now and love and accept myself as I am today.

Even though I don't feel acceptable, I choose to release this fear and feel relaxed and calm within.

Even though I just stuffed my face and I feel disgusting, I forgive myself because I'm only human and humans make mistakes.

Think you've got the hang of it? If so, let's get tapping!

3. TAP.

You will tap on a series of meridian points on your upper body while speaking aloud. Again, be sure to bring the full intensity of the negative emotion to your tapping sequence. The more you feel, the more you will release. And if you find it difficult to fully feel the pain, set your intent to feel it and release it, and just do your best. You will get the release you are ready for as you are ready for it.

The first point you will tap on is called the karate-chop point because it's the part of your hand you would use to make a karate chop. It's the fleshy part on the side of your palm, below the pinky and above the wrist. Use three fingers of your right hand to gently tap on the fleshy part of your left hand while you say your intention statement three times: *Even though weight loss is hard work, I am releasing this now and I deeply and completely love and accept myself.*

Next, repeat only the negatively charged phrase from your intention statement, the part that you want to release—*Weight loss is hard work*—and gently tap on the following points:

1. The crown of your head
2. Just above your inner eyebrows, one hand tapping either side
3. At the end of your eyebrows, beside your eyes, one hand on either side
4. The bony ridge just below your eyes, one hand on either side
5. The "mustache" space between your nose and your upper lip
6. The crease in your chin
7. Just below your clavicles (these bones run horizontally on your upper chest, just below your neck)
8. Your inner wrists or pulse points (you can just tap them together)
9. The back of your left hand on the small soft spot or indentation between the bone that runs to your pinky finger and the bone that runs to your ring finger
10. The back of your right hand in the same spot

Once you've tapped on all your meridian points, finish by tapping on the karate-chop point of your right hand while saying aloud only your positive affirmation: *I am releasing this now and I deeply and completely love and accept myself.*

Note: The Emotional Freedom Technique is especially effective when done with a partner. One person can be the guide, leading the other person through the charged emotional statements, and the other person can simply follow and feel the feelings. To do the Emotional Freedom Technique with your Full-Filled weight-release buddy, pretend you are playing the children's game "Simon Says." Explain your issue and the negative charge to your buddy. He or she will then pretend to be you and say your intention statement for you while tapping on his or her own karate-chop point. You will tap in tandem and repeat what your partner says. Your partner will then say the negative phrase and tap on all his or her meridian points, and you will follow, tapping on your own points all the way through the round.

4. TAKE A DEEP BREATH AND CHECK INSIDE.

Simply notice how you feel. Perhaps you feel energy moving around inside. Notice if any images, new thoughts, or feelings come to mind. Pay attention to what they are. Check in with the emotional charge. How does it compare to how it was before? Has it lessened? Often, releasing negative emotions with the Emotional Freedom Technique is like peeling back the layers of an onion. After you release the surface-level feelings, you may become aware of deeper emotions that are now ready to be released. Feel free to adapt your intention statement as you peel back the layers. The following is a simplified tapping sequence I might have used with the Over-achieving Multitasker from Week 2. In this example, we start tapping before she knows what her deep fear and limiting beliefs are. We start simply with what she is feeling most acutely in the moment and progress from there.

ROUND 1

Even though I feel disgusting because I just ate something I shouldn't have, I am choosing to forgive myself because I deeply and completely love and accept myself.

(By the end of Round 1, my client feels less guilty about snacking at the office and starts to focus instead on the work project she'd been avoiding by eating.)

ROUND 2

Even though I'm dreading this project, I'm choosing to feel relaxed, and I deeply and completely love and accept myself.

(By the end of Round 2, she realizes that what she's truly afraid of is failing, losing her job, and ending up on the street.)

ROUND 3

Even though I'm terrified of failing, being fired, and losing everything, I'm letting go of the root cause of this fear. I'm forgiving myself for being imperfect and choosing to deeply and completely love and accept myself.

(By the end of Round 3, the guilt she initially started tapping on is gone, and she's feeling much lighter and better about herself. She has just released a deep fear and limiting belief—that she will eventually lose everything—and in its place she has a new relaxed confidence that satisfies her craving for the old afternoon munchies. Now, that's sweet success!)

There are many ways in which you can play with the wording of the Emotional Freedom Technique, so feel free to adjust your intention statement until it feels just right. The only hard-and-fast rule to follow is that you feel the negative feelings intensely while you're tapping so that you can release them. If you don't feel them, you won't release them. Though this might be uncomfortable, the cool thing about the EFT is that as you bring up a negatively charged emotion, you are in that moment releasing it. The two happen almost simultaneously. Here are some other examples of ways to play with the wording:

Even though I am eating because I am bored, I'm open to releasing any deeper issues I may have as I easily eat to nourish a slim and healthy body.

Even though I feel sad about losing food as my best friend, I'm letting that sadness go and inviting in positive energy and a fresh perspective.

Even though it feels impossible to change because I have tried so many times before, it sure would be amazing to be naturally slim and healthy, and I invite it in.

Even though I am so afraid that I will lose my connection to my friends if I become slim, I'm letting go of that fear and choosing to have an even better connection to those closest to me as I become a slim and healthy person.

Even though I feel hopeless because I've screwed up again, I'm choosing to let my screwups make me stronger, so I'm choosing to forgive, love, and accept myself.

Even though I've always been fat, I'm letting that go now and choosing a new identity that is more authentically me, that allows me to be healthy, slim, and fit. I'm choosing a new identity that honors all of who I am and can be.

Even though I am afraid that if I get what I want something bad will happen, and I'd rather have the problems I'm familiar with, I'm releasing those old fears and beliefs and inviting in positive energy and a new, positive perspective.

Even though I am deeply afraid that if I am more successful than my parents I will lose my connection with them, I'm letting go of that fear and inviting in an even deeper, more openhearted connection with them, as I am more successful.

Even though I can't imagine who I will be if I don't have my struggle with weight and I'm scared, I'm beginning to think that it might be fun to discover the new me one day at a time!

5. REPEAT.

The EFT is best done in rounds of two or more, but feel free to do as many rounds as you like to completely release your limiting beliefs. You may feel a shift immediately or more subtly over time.

Someone Who Tried This Before You

Always known as the chubby member of her family, Sheila struggled to see herself as slim and healthy. After the breakup of her marriage, she renewed her efforts to slim down in the hope of attracting a new relationship into her life. She arrived at her session concerned about overeating at an upcoming family event.

I asked her to imagine going through the event behaving as she would like to behave, and then I asked her what was stopping her from being that way. She felt that her family expected her to eat a lot and that she would find it difficult to change given their expectations and past experiences. We then began tapping, using the EFT to help her move through this block. We started with the following phrasing:

Even though I feel pressure from my family to eat, I still deeply and completely love and accept myself.

During the tapping, Sheila began thinking about how her mother used to tell her, "Your nose is too big, your thighs are too fat, and your waist is too wide. You'll never have a boyfriend." As might anyone who'd grown up hearing such things, Sheila had come to believe that she was indeed unlovable and that that was the cause of the failure of her marriage.

We then tapped on:

Even though I am unlovable because my nose is too big, my thighs are too fat, and my waist is too wide, I still deeply and completely love and accept myself.

Saying those horrifying thoughts out loud while tapping actually got her laughing about how silly they were. Laughter is a powerful healer, and in Sheila's case, it was mixed with tears of release. By the time we finished, the notion that she was unlovable seemed ridiculous to Sheila. She left the session that day feeling quite lovable and worthy.

Another thing I love about the Emotional Freedom Technique is that you can do it on your own in the moment of distress, specifically after an overeating episode when you are in the full fury of your guilt and self-criticism. In such instances, the EFT works as a self-correction technique, effectively releasing your guilt and further deflating the cycle of overeating. Because the best time to perform the Emotional Freedom Technique is when you're experiencing an intense negative emotional charge, many of my clients have gotten into the habit of slipping out of dinners, parties, or meetings and into the restroom to do a quick round or two of tapping. They self-correct on the spot and return to the group relaxed and relieved.

Food for Thought

If you have a sincere desire and the appropriate tools, change is possible. It's not time-bound; healing can occur at any age, for anybody, in an instant. Change is possible! I don't care how much extra weight you have; I don't care how long you've been struggling. I have had clients in their sixties and seventies who have never been successful in the past finally make changes when they commit to the practices of the Full-Filled program. Their excess weight drops off, and, more important, they awaken to the rest of their lives.

When you tap immediately following a major screwup, you save yourself a lot of precious time by not wallowing in guilty feelings. Your intention sentence might sound something like this: *Even though I just stuffed my face and I feel like a hideous pig, I'm choosing to forgive, love, and accept myself.* Or *Even though I just ate way past full and feel disappointed in myself, I am choosing to let the guilt go and learn from this experience.* Or *Even though I ate when I wasn't hungry, I still choose to easily release my excess weight.*

In addition to using the Emotional Freedom Technique to self-correct on the spot, you can also use this tool as part of your Re-Do. (Remember the Re-Do from last week? It's a visualization process where you re-do your past slip-up in your mind, replacing it with an image of how you wish you had behaved instead, creating a new behavior pattern for your mind to follow in the future.) If you want to incorporate the Emotional Freedom Technique into the Re-Do before settling into the visualization process, first tap out any negative feelings associated with overeating. For example, *Even though I lost control and stuffed my face, I'm releasing my guilt and forgiving myself, because I deeply and completely love and accept myself.* Doing the Emotional Freedom Technique this way will help clear negative emotional interference and allow the Re-Do to take deeper root as a new behavior pattern that you will automatically follow the next time you're in a similar situation.

You can also incorporate the Emotional Freedom Technique into your Pre-Dos. (The Pre-Do is a Re-Do for the future instead of the past.) If you have a special restaurant party, family event, or social or work hour coming up and you are concerned about overeating, you might imagine yourself feeling and behaving the way you want to feel in that future situation and then tap on your intention statement. For example, you might say, *Even though there's not enough time to drop my excess weight before the family reunion, I deeply and completely love and accept myself.* Or *Even though I'm afraid of the judgment of those around me, I choose to let this fear go and feel good about myself.*

Someone Who Tried This Before You

The owner of a successful luxury goods business, Ilaria lived a glamorous life. She regularly dined in fine restaurants and shuttled between her homes—one in the city and the other in the country. Although she wasn't overweight, she struggled with food obsession and binge eating and came to me desperate for help.

After the first session, her overeating and food thoughts had diminished dramatically. Excited by the shift, she wanted to take it further. I taught her the Emotional Freedom Technique during the next session and recommended she use it whenever an unwanted food thought or compulsion came to her.

At our check-in a week later, she had made even more progress and was, for the first time she could remember, feeling at ease about eating. I asked her how the tapping was going.

"Oh, I've been tapping all the time," she said, and she meant it. It seemed that she had gone on a tapping binge. She tapped at home, she tapped at work, and she tapped while driving (which I definitely do not recommend and discouraged her from pursuing!), though I encouraged her to pull off the road and park whenever she felt the need to tap while driving so she could do it safely!

By our fourth session, she felt her food issues were virtually gone. She was also feeling more creative and effective in her work and happier in her life. A couple years later, she contacted me and let me know that binge eating was a distant memory and she was about to take her dream sabbatical in France!

Unconditional Self-Acceptance and Love

So why all this talk this week about self-acceptance and unconditional love? Self-acceptance and unconditional love are spiritual concepts that assert that, at our core, we are each good, deserving, and worthy. These concepts are what the Full-Filled program is really all about. In fact, unconditional self-acceptance and love form the foundation for lasting change and a fulfilling life.

Most people refuse to accept themselves as they are—flawed, "fat," imperfect human beings—because they believe that, if they do, they'll lose both their short- and long-term motivation to change and become complacent and lazy. They believe that only by being tough on themselves, and sometimes even downright hurtful and cruel, will they stay motivated towards their goal. I should know; I used to do it all the time. I pushed myself to meet extremely high standards (I was the Perfectionist type), and when I didn't meet my high standards, which was most of the time, I would treat myself terribly, wielding insults like balls from a pitching machine. All that negativity certainly had an effect—it made me work harder in many areas of my life, and I did well by external standards—but with my body it backfired. Why? Because berating myself made me feel like crap. And what was my number one feel-good trick? Eating!

Do you, too, hold yourself to extremely high standards that seem impossibly hard to meet? Is your aim to be perfect? Assuming your answer is yes, let me ask you another question. Do you know of anything that's perfect that continues to grow and change? Think about it. Does anything come to mind? Moreover, do you love anyone who's perfect? Do you even *know* anyone who's perfect?

Perfection is the antithesis of growth. Though this idea may seem backward, if you want to change your body and your life and evolve and grow into your dream self, you must accept and love your imperfect self—cellulite, flabby belly, and all—just as you are today. Research has shown that babies who have all of their physical needs met but do not receive adequate love will suffer from a condition called "failure to thrive," which can be fatal. With sufficient love, however, infants grow and change at an astounding rate. Love fuels their growth.

Love is a required ingredient for positive change. So why wouldn't the same principle apply to you? News flash: the same principle does apply to you! When you realize that accepting and loving yourself will promote rather than detract from lasting personal growth, your life will transform in more positive ways.

To deepen your unconditional self-acceptance and nurture your growth, try the following mindful meditation, "A Journey of Self-Acceptance." If any barriers or concerns come up during the process, remember that this is only an experiment to see what happens when you truly love and accept yourself just as you are. Even if you can't yet imagine feeling this good about yourself, I still encourage you to go through the process.

Mindful Meditation: A Journey of Self-Acceptance

Begin this short visualization journey by setting your intent to regard yourself as deserving of unconditional acceptance and love. Specifically, *your* unconditional acceptance and love. Next, think of someone or something that you love unconditionally. Maybe it's a child in your life or a pet. Maybe it's you as a child. Take a few moments and think of someone or something for whom you feel unbounded, unconditional love. Once you have an image in your mind of who or what that is, close your eyes and let yourself feel those wonderful feelings of unconditional acceptance and love. Feel your heart open and your love pour out for that being, that creature, that person. Experience the fullness of your acceptance. Revel in your feelings of love. Notice those feelings as you look at that being. What a delight it is to accept and love someone or something in this way!

Next, create in your mind's eye an image of yourself. Notice how different you feel about yourself! Now I want you to see yourself in the same way that you just saw this image of your beloved. Take your time. If transferring those feelings of acceptance and love onto yourself isn't working, go back to the image of your beloved and feel the good feelings you have towards him or her.

Now swap out the image of your beloved with your own image by putting yourself in the same place in your inner visual field. For example, if you imagined your beloved from just the shoulders up, imagine yourself from just the shoulders up. If you saw your beloved in a beautiful light, see yourself in the same light. See yourself in exactly the same way. You will know you are successful when you feel the same kind and loving feelings towards yourself as you feel towards your beloved. Again, take your time with this.

Allow those good feelings about yourself to wander through your dreams tonight, and tomorrow morning, when you look into the bathroom mirror, look deep into your own eyes and notice what comes up. Beyond the physical, do you see something deeper there—a being who is both vulnerable and imperfect and beautiful and deserving of your acceptance and love simply because he or she exists?

A client of mine named Gabby had great success with this meditation when she focused on an old photo of herself as a young child. She said, "When I look at this old photo of me, I'm filled with so much love and admiration for this little girl. She has been my most faithful friend and constant companion. She has dealt with so many things and survived them. She is beautiful and trusting, strong, resilient. I just love her.

"Reflecting on this image gave me not only amazing insights into my own strength and resilience, but peace with the idea that that child had done the best that she could throughout her life with all that she had encountered. How can I possibly be mad at her? How can I do anything but love and be grateful to and for her? When I think of her smiling and beaming, I'm nearly brought to tears.

"I swapped out that image with one of me this morning as I took one final glance in the mirror before heading to work. The practice of bringing the love and acceptance that I feel for little me to the current me is an absolutely joyous blessing."

What would it be like if you saw yourself every day in the same way in which you regard the person or being you already love unconditionally and wholeheartedly? Can you imagine what that would feel like? How your life might change?

Most overeaters think their essence is bad and that's why their behavior is bad. I used to think that about myself, too, but it's simply not true. Your essence is not bad. Your essence is good, divine, and beautiful. Accept it. And when you do, when you accept yourself as "good," as someone worthy of love and care, the nasty, negative talk that's been hogging your airwaves for years will fade away. Once the self-hatred falls away, an even more astonishing thing happens: you will discover a reservoir of compassion and kindness for yourself you didn't think you had, and you will actually want to start treating yourself better. Nurturing self-care will become a big *yes* in your life!

Someone Who Tried This Before You

Annie had a very active inner critic and became aware of how active it was only after we started working together. She realized that she spent the majority of her days caught up in self-criticism.

"How's the tough-love approach working out for you?" I asked.

"Not good," she said. "My critical voice makes me feel awful about myself."

Annie's critical voice was beating her down, making her weak, and, as a result, leading her directly back to food in the classic cycle of overeating: feel bad → eat to feel good → feel bad for overeating → eat to feel better. She wanted to know how she could turn down the volume on her critical inner voice and break the cycle.

I said, "Let's think about this inner critic of yours. What do you suppose is the positive intent of your critic?" Annie had to really think about this. Her inner critic was so negative that she had a hard time thinking that there was anything positive about it. Finally, she said, "I guess it's trying to make me better. It wants me to be a better, more successful person."

I said, "Assuming this is true, instead of trying to silence your inner critic, what if you thanked it for how much it cares about you and wants to help you?"

Annie was a little skeptical but left the session after pledging to give it a try. Not soon after, I received the following e-mail from her:

"Becoming aware of my inner critic and defusing his bluster with a simple 'thank you' has completely rocked my relationship with him. It's exciting. The whole concept has reminded me of a Bible story. In the Old Testament, Genesis, Jacob wrestles an angel in the desert. When I read and studied this story in college, I loved it because it reminded me of my own struggles with my inner demons.

"This morning on my run, I thought about how my inner critic is like the angel in that story, and about how I wrestle with him on most days, and what would happen if I chose not to wrestle, and instead express gratitude to him for coming when I call and for working overtime to meet my requests? When I think about it like that, he's doing a fantastic job!

"This morning, I realized that my inner critic is particularly loud and active in the morning. While running is extremely cathartic for me, I noticed that it's also when my critic shouts at me the loudest and when I shout back. So this morning I decided to try the new approach of gratitude. I must have thanked my critic thirty times throughout my run. I also visualized myself in the desert and I imagined my inner critic as an angel, and as he approached me, I thanked him for showing up. When he tried wrestling with me, I didn't fight back. I sat on the desert floor peacefully, exuding love and gratitude. This visualization swept me with a sense of calm, and all of a sudden I stopped wrestling in my mind. And instead, I was free to enjoy the beauty of my morning run."

By not engaging in the usual shouting match with her inner critic and expressing gratitude instead, Annie started to feel much better about herself, and that gave rise to an innate desire to nurture and care for herself. (We naturally want to take care of the people we love.) The first thing that shifted was her attitude towards exercise. Whereas before she had often run as punishment for overeating and her excess weight, she started to enjoy it more than ever. Next, she noticed that her voracious appetite disappeared. She no longer needed food in the way she had before to fill up her energy reserves. Unconditional love and self-acceptance became the fuel that energized her and allowed her to create new, healthful, and long-lasting behaviors.

Unconditional self-acceptance and love are the foundation for lasting behavior change to take root and grow. Remember that garden we've been talking about? Unconditional self-acceptance and love is like Miracle-Gro; it fertilizes the soil to create a healthy root system, fast growth, and abundant life. When you accept and love yourself for who you are today, your life will take off, blossom, and thrive as never before. You might find that you eat more healthfully, sleep more, engage more with those around you, and move your body in ways that leave you feeling energized, not sluggish and stuffed. And that's not all. The topper on the low-fat cake is that all this acceptance and self-love will enable you to release significant amounts of weight. Who knew?

If this sounds like the breakthrough moment you've been waiting for, it is! Are you able to digest what I'm saying? You can actually love yourself slim and healthy. Not the approach you're used to, right? As I was, you're probably more familiar with the hate-yourself-thin method. How's it been working for you? I tried it more than a few times, and it sucked me right into a deep, dark pit of self-loathing. Human beings prefer feeling good to feeling bad any day of the week, which makes the unconditional love approach so much more enjoyable. Plus, it actually works!

Food for Thought

Once you accept yourself as you are now, the natural consequence is wanting to take wonderful care of yourself. Then it's a very simple matter to add behaviors such as eating good food and engaging in activities that nourish and invigorate your body. Unconditional self-acceptance is the foundation on which all behavior change is built. Until you have that foundation, any changes in behavior that you make will be willpower-based and will not last.

Can you imagine loving yourself so much that you feel an overwhelming desire to take the very best care of yourself you possibly can? I've seen clients transform before my very eyes after they make the switch from self-hatred to self-acceptance and love. It's as if, all of a sudden, their loving spirit shines out from behind their eyes. With the cycle of self-criticism and abuse broken, they're free. And with this new freedom is a readiness and eagerness to share that acceptance and love with other people. When you come from a place of acceptance, love, peace, and fulfillment, you have more to give the world. The positive effects of accepting and loving yourself ripple outward, and they're considerable. Imagine if all the self-hating overeaters in the world stopped hating themselves and started accepting and loving themselves. Now, that would be a revolution!

Food for Thought

Why does losing weight matter? It matters not so much in the "I'm getting ready for swimsuit season" kind of way or the "I'm getting ready for my high school reunion" kind of way but rather in the "Live your life to the fullest" kind of way. Your weight struggle has been holding you back from who you can be in the world. Let releasing the struggle free you to truly enjoy the rest of your life and generously share the gifts of your authentic self.

I regularly run through Golden Gate Park in San Francisco, and when I do, I often pass a man whom I can only describe as a joyous character. He looks like a cross between a musician and a slightly scruffy shaman with his shock of gray-black hair and beard. Without fail, he greets everyone he passes in the park with a genuine "Hello!" accompanied by an ear-to-ear grin. I tend to be a bit inward when I run. I don't make a lot of eye contact with people or feel comfortable extending my energy out to others, but whenever I see this guy beaming at me as I pass, I'm pulled out of my introverted state. I simply can't resist his joy. It's that big. In fact, on a number of occasions we've exchanged a high five (which is not something I typically do with characters on the street)! But the simple presence of this guy is an energy booster, and that's because he's emanating unadulterated love. It's almost as though you can see him glowing from within and radiating his positive energy outward to others. It's an amazing thing to witness and a huge gift. It certainly makes my day!

How might your life change if you accepted and loved yourself as that man does? If you were full on the inside, how might it manifest on the outside? Think about that as you ease into the following mindful meditation, "Gratitude and Manifestation."

Mindful Meditation: Gratitude and Manifestation

Sit in a comfortable place where you can easily relax. Focus on your breath, and take several deep breaths in and out. Turn your attention and awareness to the base of your body, and begin to imagine a cord or root extending out of the base of your body. Imagine it extending down through the floor, into the earth, and reaching deep and wide much like a root system that would support a tall and majestic tree that sways gently to the winds and storms of life.

Each time you exhale, imagine any stress or toxins releasing down through your root system and into the cool earth, where they are composted and recycled into nutrient-rich soil.

As you inhale, feel the nourishment from the earth travel up through your body, renewing you and nourishing your soul and spirit. Feel this positive pure energy travel all the way up into your heart space. Repeat this exercise for a few minutes, enjoying the renewing properties and nourishment you gather from the earth.

Next, imagine an opening at the top of your head. Visualize a column of beautiful light traveling down from the sky and descending into the crown of your head. Feel the light descend through your head and down through your shoulders and upper chest and into your heart space. This light brings with it imagination, insight, and creativity, and in your heart space it mixes with the nourishing and stabilizing energy provided by the earth. The light energy inspires change, while the earth energy manifests change on the material plane. The energies meet, mix, and mingle in your heart space, and as they do, they open and expand your heart. As your heart energy continues to open and expand, it radiates outward to the world around you, carrying with it your heart's desires.

Notice how this beautiful heart energy carries with it both a profound gratitude for the present and excitement for the future. You are supported and inspired by your heart's desires. Revel in these positive feelings and notice your heart opening even more, supplying you with an abundance of loving energy for you to freely share with the world.

When you feel ready, come back fully into your body in the present moment, awake, aware, and alert, feeling refreshed and renewed.

The true reward of accepting and loving yourself for who you are today is that it releases and frees up all the energy and time you've spent obsessing over food and lost in negative self-talk. You see, every minute you spend tangled up in criticism and unhappy with yourself is a minute lost from your life. Once you're free, you will get back what feels like an endless amount of time to rediscover who you are. And you do know by now that your size does not define you, right? You're much more than what you eat and weigh. You have beautiful gifts and talents to offer the world around you, and once you've turned down the voice of your inner critic and resolved the pain underneath your weight struggle, there will be nothing stopping you from sharing your light with the world. This was your life's purpose all along, not hitting a low number on the scale.

When I was still stuck in the weight struggle, I had no idea who I was other than "Hi, my name is Renée, and I'm a freak around food." It was only after I confronted my fear of inadequacy, changed my limiting beliefs about success, and accepted myself for who I was that I discovered my true passion and purpose in life: to help people like you end your struggle with weight and discover your true gifts.

 Food for Thought

Go ahead and explore your unique gifts in the safety of your imagination. Take hidden glances at them while waiting in the checkout line or stopped at traffic lights. Let your mind go while you're lathering up in the shower or lifting weights in the gym. Contemplate the gifts you have to offer the world. Big or small, how might you express them? Have fun. Enjoy the discovery.

In the absence of the consuming weight struggle, clients of mine have repurposed their newfound energy in a variety of ways to bring joy and fullness to their lives. One went back to school to get a degree in sustainable business; another created a nonprofit to help poor women start artisanal food businesses; a third, who, when we began working together, had been terrified of riding a public bus for fear of being ridiculed for her size, traveled alone to Europe and Africa. Another client, who was twice divorced from abusive men, finally met and married a loving and wonderful man who likes to start his day by telling her how beautiful she is. Another ended a seven-year relationship that she realized was going nowhere and is happier now more than ever being single and free. What you do with your new self and energy doesn't really matter. It could be grand, minimal, or something in between. What does matter is that whatever it is, it lights you up because whatever lights you up will benefit everyone who comes into contact with you. That's when you'll know your life is finally yours again.

Progress Report

Over the next seven days, be sure to:

1. **Identify and catalog your trigger foods and trigger situations in your Full-Filled Weight-Release Journal.** Your triggers are the most direct, effective way to get to the root of any unhealed pain that's holding you back, so list the situations that come up the most frequently and that, 90 percent of the time, cause you to head face-first into the food. Also, list your worst trigger foods—changing your compulsion to eat these to a take-it-or-leave-it attitude would make the biggest positive difference in your life.

2. **Identify and catalog your limiting beliefs.** Your limiting beliefs support your unresolved fears that drive you to overeat. Ask yourself, "Where does this fear come from? What core limiting beliefs do I have that support this fear?" Record your limiting beliefs in your Full-Filled Weight-Release Journal.

3. **Change your limiting beliefs into new, empowering beliefs.** The way to change a limiting belief is by introducing doubt through questioning or humor. After you question and introduce doubt to your old beliefs, start looking for and writing down counter-examples to your beliefs in your Full-Filled Weight-Release Journal. Replace your limiting beliefs with empowering beliefs that you state in the present and in the positive. Try your new, empowering beliefs on for size and refine them until they feel just right.

4. **Use the Emotional Freedom Technique to release your limiting beliefs and instill your new, empowering beliefs.** After you begin the work of transforming your old, limiting beliefs into empowering beliefs, it's important to release the emotional hold

that your old beliefs have on you. To release the negative feelings and thoughts associated with your limiting beliefs, use the Emotional Freedom Technique and replace them with positive ones. Practice the EFT at least twice this week, and increase your use of the technique in the upcoming weeks to as much as once a day.

5. **Think about the unique gifts you have to offer the world.** Once you've transformed your beliefs and resolved the pain underneath your weight struggle, there's nothing stopping you from sharing your light with the world. Contemplate the gifts you have to offer the world. Big or small, how might you express them?

The Secret of Easy, Pleasurable Eating

Over the past four weeks of the Full-Filled program, you've had many breakthrough moments and made significant progress by clearing your inner objections, discovering the gifts you've been trying to get from food, transforming your limiting beliefs into empowering beliefs, and releasing the pain that's been holding you back from becoming your dream self. Now, with a rich foundation of forgiveness, acceptance, and self-love beneath you, you're set up for monumental behavior change like you haven't seen yet. I'm talking about changes that affect when, how much, and what you eat on a daily basis.

Maybe you're thinking it's about time. We've gone four weeks without any specific mention of food. You're right, and that's because the secret to becoming slim and healthy for a lifetime has much more to do with how you think and feel about yourself than it does with strict adherence to a magical fat-burning food plan.

Most diet programs have it backward. They jump in with eating-behavior change from page one. They spend a great deal of time telling you what to eat and little if any time helping you figure out how on earth you're going to stick to their eating plan longer than your current burst of resolve. Most diet and weight loss books don't acknowledge that reliable and lasting physical change is an inside job. Thankfully, you know this now. You've spent the last four weeks doing that deep internal work, and now you're ready to turn that progress inside out.

In Week 5 of the Full-Filled program, you will learn:

- The naturally slim and healthy mind-set
- How to tune in to your body's cues and change your cravings
- Why eating for pleasure takes the pounds off
- How structure and routine can give you freedom
- The steps to reinvigorate your motivation to exercise

What's Their Trick?

As you begin Week 5 of the Full-Filled program, **set your intention to change your mind-set about hunger and begin to prefer eating in a way that will give you the most pleasure for the longest time**. Take a deep, cleansing breath and set your intention now.

When it comes to what and when to eat, the Full-Filled program is based on the mind-set of naturally slim and healthy people—you know, the ones who, year after year, eat what they want, leave food on their plates, and never seem to go up and down in weight. We love to hate them because we believe we can never be like them. Not true.

Contrary to popular belief, being naturally slim and healthy often has little if nothing to do with good genes, a fast metabolism, or strong willpower. Simply put, naturally slim and healthy people consistently and effortlessly make good decisions about what and how they eat because they have a good decision-making strategy that listens to their body's natural cues and maximizes pleasure. Yes— naturally slim and healthy people eat for pleasure! Imagine that, and know that you, too, can implement this strategy and experience similar results. All it requires is that you learn to think as they do, which is something you already know how to do: you change your mind-set so that you can easily change your behaviors. That's what you've been practicing for several weeks now.

Think for a moment about a naturally slim and healthy person. You probably know someone like that—a relative, parent, sibling, cousin, or maybe your BFF or a coworker you see every day. Those are the people you look at and wonder, "No matter what they eat, they always seem to be slim and healthy. Maintaining their ideal weight does not appear to be a struggle for them. How do they do it?"

Back when I was struggling with my obsessive-compulsive eating habits, I, too, was baffled and often annoyed at how some people could eat just one cookie or a few bites of cake—and stop. Back then, I was a card-carrying member of the clean-plate club, and I knew when to stop eating sweets—when they were all gone! I longed to get into the heads of the skinny and really understand how they ate that way, and especially how they seemed to do it so easily. Yet no matter how many slimming secrets I read about or how many diet and nutrition books I consumed, I could never figure it out. To me, they were simply an alien species!

If you, too, have convinced yourself that naturally slim and healthy people are just a freaky group of metabolic superbeings (to which you don't belong), let me break the good news to you: nothing could be further from the truth. The naturally slim and healthy don't meticulously count calories, carbohydrate grams, and fat grams, nor do they follow a magic formula that says something like "Never mix a protein with a fruit past six o'clock on a full moon." In fact, I bet the average naturally slim and healthy person in many places in the world doesn't even know what a protein gram is.

If they aren't nutritional experts and they don't practice an underground form of alchemy, what's their trick? How do they eat what they want and so easily maintain their weight—a feat that for the rest of us seems to require either physical restraint or an act of God to achieve?

Their trick is that they have a very simple, intuitive eating strategy. "Simple" is key. If it weren't—if it required the hard work and diligence we often think it does—do you think they'd be able to stick to it and keep their weight off year after year? No, because when staying slim and healthy means deprivation and endless effort, the weight eventually piles back on. Ninety-nine percent of people who lose weight will regain it within five years. When stress comes up in our lives—changing jobs, starting or ending a relationship, suffering a financial strain—we're more likely than not to throw discipline out the window and go back to our old ways. Given those discouraging odds, in order to be successful, you need a weight-release plan that's easy to follow and maintain, and that's exactly what the naturally slim and healthy have discovered.

"So," you ask, "how do they do it, Renée?" Naturally slim and healthy people maintain their weight by—wait for it—matching their calorie intake with their calorie burn rate. The formula is very simple: calories in equals calories out equals weight stability. Fewer calories in and more calories out equals release. More calories in than calories out equals gain. That's it. That's how the naturally slim and healthy decide how much and what to eat.

I apologize if this isn't the big Aha! moment you were waiting for, but there is no secret formula or magic pill to being slim. It comes down to a very simple calculation: match the calories you eat to the calories you burn, and you will maintain your weight. Consume less than you burn, and you will lose weight. Consume more than you burn, and you'll store the extra calories as fat and gain weight. It sounds easy enough, except for the inconvenient fact that most of us want to eat more than we burn.

Many people, and maybe this includes you, believe that their weight challenges result from a slow metabolism and that naturally slim and healthy people must have a high metabolism that vaporizes everything they eat before it can turn into fat. Again, not true. Anyone can be naturally slim and healthy, no matter what his or her metabolism is. The challenge is not how fast or slow your system runs; it's your desire and propensity to eat more than your body requires. If you want to lose weight, you must eat less than what you burn. Period.

Now you may be wondering, "How on earth can I know how many calories I burn, so I can eat less than that number and lose weight without spending big bucks on the latest metabolism-measuring gadget or expensive testing? And furthermore, what does any of this have to do with pleasure?" We'll get to pleasure in a moment, but in reply to your first question: the answer is hunger. Yes, hunger, not some fancy gadget you strap to your arm. Hunger is what the naturally slim and healthy use to match their intake with their burn rate. Specifically designed by Mother Nature herself and included in the standard equipment of the human body, hunger succinctly and accurately tells us when we need more food and when we've had enough. By tuning in to your body and paying close attention to your physical hunger, you can easily match your calorie intake to your calorie burn rate and become naturally slim and healthy for a lifetime.

Get Hungry

Before you start thinking, "Wait a minute, I don't know if I can do that" or "Maybe I didn't get the standard equipment," let's take a few minutes to discuss hunger in general. It's very common for people who struggle with their weight to feel panicky around hunger, and this fear is endlessly perpetuated by the diet industry. Fasts, detox diets, and weight loss plans proudly make claims such as "Never be hungry again" or "Eliminate hunger forever," pushing the idea that hunger is something we should either ignore or avoid at all costs. Indeed, many of my first-time clients come to me with "hunger phobia," convinced that hunger is a bad and very scary thing.

Angela, an *Inside Out Weight Loss* podcast listener, successfully lost about 70 pounds following my program. When she was explaining some of the shifts she had experienced on her weight-release journey, she shared how she used to react to hunger and likened it to a fear of getting shot. "I know this sounds dramatic," Angela said, "but it's almost as if you're thinking to yourself, 'I better put my bulletproof vest on before that awful hunger comes to get me!'" What most scared Angela about hunger was her emotional reaction to it. Once she was able to let go of her fear (after a few renewing rounds of the Emotional Freedom Technique) and realize that hunger is just a temporary, passing physical feeling indicating a need for nourishment, she learned to look forward to it.

You see, hunger doesn't have to be a high-drama event; it's actually a really great thing. In fact, it's an extraordinary tool and one you want to cultivate, nurture, and appreciate. It's the best feedback system there is to let you know what your body's needs are for optimal health. It tells you if you've eaten the right amount of food, it tells you if you've had too much, and it tells you if you need more food during a meal. Hunger helps you better than any technology designed to date, and it's completely free! There's no good reason not to use it!

This week, you will work on reacquainting yourself with your hunger. I'm not talking about fall-on-the-floor, I'm-going-to-pass-out-because-my-blood-sugar-is-so-low hunger, but the kind of hunger that says, "Hey, my stomach is getting empty. Soon it will be time for some food" or "My stomach is starting to feel full and satisfied. It's time to put down my fork and push away my plate." Tuning in to your hunger makes it very easy to keep your intake and burn rate effectively in check.

Food for Thought

I'll tell you a secret: it is very, very rare for a person to be overweight if she eats when she's physically hungry. The majority of people who are overweight are not overweight because they eat when they are hungry. They are overweight because they eat when they are *not* truly physically hungry or eat past the point of being full.

Tuning in to your hunger doesn't mean you're going to starve yourself, so before the warning bells go off, signaling strict discipline and deprivation, take a deep breath. All you're going to do is learn to tune in to your body and appreciate the feeling of hunger so that you can manage your food intake in a way that's easy and nonthreatening.

Tuning Into Your Hunger

Ask yourself, "How tuned in to physical hunger am I? How tuned in to my physical body am I?" If your answer is "I don't feel connected or tuned in," know that you're not alone. If you feel as if you're never truly hungry or as if you're always hungry, you're also in good company.

Let's first address why you might never feel hungry. There are two good reasons. The first is that you may be eating so much that your body never has an opportunity to get hungry. You may be doing this on purpose, or you may be doing it by accident. (Whichever is the case, after the deep-healing work you did last week to release your trigger situations, you're probably overeating less.) The other reason that you may never get hungry is that you've decided to turn off to the feelings of your body. In other words, you've disconnected. Many people who struggle with their weight have disconnected from their bodies and ignored hunger for so long that they don't know what hunger feels like. The reasons for this vary, but more often than not, you may have decided or felt that being in your body was painful. You may even feel that your body has betrayed you by not responding to the different diets and weight loss plans you've tried in the past. If your body has been a source of pain, discomfort, or frustration for you, it's likely that you made a decision, probably unconsciously, to tune out and not pay attention to it. (Trauma survivors, such as those who have suffered physical or sexual abuse, typically fall into this category. A gentle and healing trauma-release meditation is available on my website, www.insideoutweightloss .com.)

On the other end of the spectrum, you may have the sensation that you're always hungry. Though this is less common, people who experience constant nagging hunger often confuse physical hunger with emotional hunger. It may feel exactly the same to them, and because they're always feeling hungry, they're always eating. If you've been eating to satisfy an emotional hunger, distinguishing it from physical hunger may feel hard for you. But again, as you release the emotional pain associated with your unhealthful eating habits, reconnecting and tuning back in to your body's natural signals of hunger and satiety will become easier and easier, especially with the tools and techniques you'll learn in this week of the Full-Filled program.

 Food for Thought

If you've ever been on a strict diet or even a fast and suffered through extreme hunger, holding on just long enough to fit back into your skinny jeans or your wedding dress, you're probably less than excited about the idea of letting yourself get hungry. In fact, you may have inadvertently created a phobia or a desperate fear of hunger.

Check inside, and if fear of hunger is something that is operating within you, you'll especially enjoy learning how to adjust your appetite and rebuild your relationship with hunger pangs. The Emotional Freedom Technique is a great way to release hunger phobia. Experiment with a sequence like this:

Even though I hate getting hungry because it feels like I'm going to die, I'm releasing my fear of hunger and choosing instead to enjoy hunger because it means I'm on track and will thoroughly enjoy my next meal.

The Hunger Diary

I'd like to share with you an invaluable tool that will allow you to start tuning back in to your body so that you can more easily pick up on your body's natural cues. It's called a hunger diary, which is a variation of a food diary, a tool that many nutritionists use, except that instead of documenting what you eat, you will be monitoring your body's hunger cues and tracking how hungry you are before and after every meal. Though research shows that food diaries work at helping curb food intake, as long as you keep them, you may negatively associate them with restriction, control, and not measuring up. If that is the case for you, please know that this is not a food diary but rather a hunger diary. Also, know that keeping a hunger diary is not meant to be a long-term practice. It is a training tool to help you reawaken to your body's natural signals.

How it works: in your Full-Filled Weight-Release Journal, on a scale of 0 to 10, rate your hunger right before and right after you eat. Zero is famished, fall-on-the-floor hungry; 5 is neutral—you're neither hungry nor full; and 10 is "I am stuffed like a turkey on Thanksgiving Day." Most naturally slim and healthy people tend to eat when they're at 1 to 2 on the hunger scale and stop at 4 to 6. That may seem low to you, but naturally slim and healthy people like to get good and hungry before eating and then stop eating before their stomachs begin to feel full. Rarely do they say, "I think I could fit more in, so I'll keep eating until I can't swallow another bite." Eating within the 4-to-6 range increases their enjoyment of what they eat and leaves them feeling good in their bodies for the rest of the day and throughout the night.

That said, I think it's important that you set your own goal and find your own way; I don't want to dictate what number on the hunger scale you should start at or eat to. Just reduce from where you are now. So if you now begin eating when you're at a 4, start waiting to eat until you're at a 2, and see how you feel. If you've been eating up to a 9 on the hunger scale, stop eating at a 6 or 7. You likely will find this easier than you think because of the prep work you've done over the past month. This approach lends itself to continuous improvement and allows you to adjust your hunger/fullness level as your weight changes. (Depending on your weight, height, and build, weight release will most easily happen when you begin and stop eating within the 0-to-5 hunger range. You probably want to avoid getting to 0 on the hunger scale, but you might want to do it a couple times just to prove to yourself that you do, in fact, survive to tell the tale and that hunger is just a feeling.)

To determine where on the hunger scale you tend to fall and to help refamiliarize yourself with what true hunger feels like, dig into the exercise below. You will want to get into the habit of following these easy steps before and after every meal.

Dig In: Rate and Track Your Hunger

Right before and after you eat, take a moment to rate your hunger. Put your hands on your stomach and check in with your body to see how you feel. (Note that the stomach is right below your rib cage, on the left side of your body. Many people think the stomach is in the belly. It's actually above the belly.) Ask yourself, "How does my stomach feel right now?" Tilt your head down, close your eyes, and notice the physical feeling in your stomach.

Ask yourself, "Do I feel pass-out-on-the-floor hungry, stuffed-like-a-Thanksgiving-turkey full, or somewhere in between?" Rate your hunger before eating in your Full-Filled Weight-Release Journal. After you've eaten, put your hands on your stomach, check in again, and think to yourself, "Hmm, how full am I?"

If you want to lose weight, you ideally want to go into a meal feeling at 0 to 2 on the hunger scale and finish your meal at no higher than 5 to 6. Eating within this range may take a while for you to get used to, so take it slowly and be easy on yourself. Your first order of business is simply to get into a habit of noticing your hunger and when you typically eat.

Below is a sample hunger diary table that many of my clients use, with a bonus column to help you focus on how food feels in your body over time. We'll be talking about the importance of this extra column in a minute. (An electronic hunger diary form is available for free at my website, www.insideoutweightloss.com.)

Hunger Diary

0 = starving ➜ 10 = stuffed

Date	Time	Food	Hunger Before Eating	Hunger After Eating	How did this food make me feel *over the next couple of hours?*

Create a table similar to this and track your hunger in your Full-Filled Weight-Release Journal. If you don't have your journal with you every time you eat, track your hunger in a small notebook you carry around in your pocket or purse, or note it in your smartphone and transfer the information into your weight-release journal later. Keeping a mental record is harder to track and less reliable, so I advise against it. If you are a visual person, you might want to graph your hunger throughout the day. Aim to keep a hunger diary for the rest of the six-week program or until you feel as though you are automatically managing your intake with your burn rate.

By tracking your hunger levels throughout the day, you will begin to notice patterns that reveal when you eat (for example, do you eat at regular mealtimes or at random times throughout the day?), situations in which you eat when you are not very hungry, and circumstances in which you stop when you are way past full. Pay attention to those patterns and the unresolved triggers that may go along with them. As you learned last week, triggers are helpful pointers to areas of yourself that still need healing work. With a little practice and an investment in identifying and releasing any remaining trigger situations, the hunger diary will help you realign your eating with your body's natural cues of hunger and satiety.

 Food for Thought

Imagine spending a cold day outdoors when you aren't wearing quite enough clothing to keep you warm. After no time at all, you become chilled to the bone, yet when you come inside, someone offers you a glass of ice water. No, thanks! You're headed straight for a long soak in a hot bath. Now imagine a hot summer day. You've been working outside and sweating away. You're absolutely parched, and someone offers you that tall glass of ice water. Heaven! Same glass of ice water, two very different experiences.

Now imagine how much you enjoy your favorite foods when you've built up a good appetite and when you take the time to really enjoy what's on your plate. Compare that with stuffing that same food down into an already full stomach. What do you prefer?

Note: If you have a strong aversion to tracking your hunger, use the Emotional Freedom Technique to release your objections or fears. Here's a sample sequence:

Even though I hate writing down my hunger because it feels like punishment and control, I'm letting go of these old associations, forgiving myself, and choosing to truly enjoy eating according to my body's needs.

Someone Who Tried This Before You

After keeping a hunger diary for a few weeks, Jane reported that her soup-and-salad lunch combo had dramatically changed. Her usual routine at lunchtime was to pile her salad plate high, fill her soup bowl to the brim, and finish both before getting up to leave. Once she started tracking her hunger, she soon discovered how much she'd been overeating. After finishing just her salad, she realized that she was already at 4 to 5 on the hunger scale, so she decided to back off her intake a bit by eating just half a bowl of soup and leaving the rest. Even then she realized she was eating more than she was truly hungry for. "No wonder the weight had piled on," she said. "Even though I've been eating healthy food, I've been eating way more than my body needs or even wants." Eventually she started ordering a simple salad and skipping the soup altogether because that's all her body needed to feel satisfied.

Rating and tracking your hunger go hand in hand with a concept I learned from the Japanese culture. You've probably noticed that Japanese people are generally pretty slim (except for those who have adopted Western ways of eating). The Japanese practice an eating strategy called *hari hachi bu*, which, literally translated, means "belly eight parts." Roughly translated, it means to eat until your belly is eight-tenths full, always leaving two-tenths space in the belly after your meal. (Mind you, eating to eight-tenths full for the Japanese is like eating to 5 or 6 on the Western hunger scale because we're used to eating large quantities. Americans eat off serving platters, whereas the Japanese feast on bite-size works of art. In many instances, it's the presentation of the food that's most fulfilling!) The Japanese practice *hari hachi bu* because they believe it maximizes enjoyment, satisfaction, and good health, and they're absolutely right.

Face it, feeling too full or stuffed feels awful. Think back to the last time you ate past full. How did you feel physically? How did those feelings affect your energy level? Your sense of well-being? Overeating makes us feel physically uncomfortable, weighted down, bloated, and sluggish. Add to that the guilt most of us stack on top of our physical discomfort for being "bad," and you have a recipe for misery. Not very appetizing!

Now think of a time when you ate when you were very hungry. When do you enjoy eating more—when you eat when you're already full or satisfied or when you eat when you're really hungry? I enjoy eating more when I'm good and hungry and I can sit down and relax in a nice setting and enjoy myself. The Japanese are the same way. They understand that high-enjoyment eating involves consuming smaller portions, appreciating the presentation and flavor of the food they're eating, and savoring each bite slowly and mindfully.

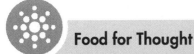

Food for Thought

The objective of tracking your hunger is to tune in to your body and learn more about it. If you forget to track and worry that you have "blown it," remember, this is a learning process. Just as in meditation, when stray thoughts appear that take you off your focus, simply notice them and bring yourself back to tracking. In fact, I recommend you do a Pre-Do of hunger tracking: imagine yourself noting your hunger before and after eating in the days and weeks ahead, until it becomes automatic. The key to success is self-correction and persistence.

The psychologist Gay Hendricks, in the movie *The Inner Weigh*, tells a story of when he first started tuning into his body rather than his emotional hunger. He was obese at the time, and he sat down at a table on which there were some blueberries. He savored and enjoyed one blueberry, then another, then a third. After finishing the third blueberry, he realized that was all his body actually needed. He was shocked! His body had so much stored energy in the form of fat that his real appetite was actually quite small. He went on to lose 120 pounds by choosing to eat only when it fed his true hunger rather than his emotional hunger.

Think about your stomach for a moment and about your feelings of hunger and satisfaction as you slip into the following mindful meditation, "The Appetite Adjuster."

Mindful Meditation: The Appetite Adjuster

At times your stomach is hungry; at other times it is satisfied. Even if you don't experience those feelings very often, you may remember experiencing them. Perhaps you can recall, or imagine, a time when you were very young, a baby perhaps, when you ate when you were hungry and stopped when you were satisfied. You stopped easily, triggering a wave of warm contentment, knowing that all was well.

When you were a baby, it was as if there was a switch inside you. When you were hungry and needed food, the switch was turned on, and you ate. When there was enough food in your body to meet your needs, the switch automatically turned off and that wave of warm contentment passed over you. Real hunger turned on the switch, and satisfaction turned it off.

You were born with that switch in you, and it's still there. In an adult body, when working properly, this switch automatically turns on and off to create a naturally slim and healthy body. It's programmed for good health and vitality. Notice this switch in you, perhaps in your torso, and notice what condition it's in. It hasn't been working very well for some time now, and you can see why. Perhaps there is clutter around the switch. Is it dirty? Has it been broken in any way? Can you move it easily from one position to the other, or has it been blocked in some way?

Now it's time to get it back into working order. Imagine clearing away all dirt, clutter, or anything else blocking the functionality of your hunger switch. Notice that it feels good to clear all that away. Perhaps you want to replace any worn or broken parts with new ones. If so, go ahead and do so.

When you have finished clearing away all the clutter, look at the switch. Notice that clearly printed on the switch are the words "on" and "off." Flip the switch a few times to test it, and make any final adjustments so that it's working perfectly, just as it did when you were a baby. Notice that only an empty stomach will turn the switch on. As long as your body has enough nourishment to be slim and healthy, the switch will remain off. Each time the switch turns off, it triggers a wave of warm contentment that washes over your body. You are neither hungry nor full but satisfied.

Now imagine what it will be like having this switch working

today, tomorrow, and the day after that, perfectly attuned to your body's natural cues of hunger and satisfaction and creating a slim and healthy body.

The Naturally Slim and Healthful Eating Strategy

So you want to eat when you're hungry—period—and you want to stop way before you are full. Remember, in order to lose weight your calorie intake must be less than your calorie output. If you eat when you're not hungry, you're consuming calories your body doesn't need. And you know what your body does with additional, unnecessary calories, right? It stores them on your backside! The key difference between how someone who overeats decides what and how much to eat and how a naturally slim and healthy person decides is that the overeater decides what to eat based on instant gratification, the feeling for the thirty seconds or minute that he or she is actively eating the food. The decision strategy for choosing what and how much to eat usually goes something like this:

1. See food.
2. Eat it.

or

1. Imagine what would taste great in your mouth in this instant.
2. Find that food or whatever is closest to it.
3. Eat it.

or

1. See food.
2. Imagine how great it would feel in your mouth while you are eating it.
3. Eat it.

Any decision process that is based solely on taste or a mouth experience (a "party in your mouth," as one client called it), in a society where tasty food is available almost everywhere at almost any time and where we're conditioned to clean our plates, will result in a lot of overeating and subsequent weight gain.

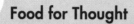

Food for Thought

When there is a mismatch between your decision strategy and the results you want, you have a recurrent problem. By adjusting your decision strategy to match the results you want, you will consistently and automatically create the results you want.

A naturally slim and healthy person, on the other hand, will decide what to eat based on true hunger and lasting gratification: the way the food will make her feel over time for the several hours that the food is being actively digested in her body. When deciding what to eat, she will ask herself questions such as:

1. Will eating this food leave me feeling energized or lethargic?
2. How will it feel in my stomach over the next couple of hours? Like a rock? Light? Satisfying?
3. Will eating this make me feel better or worse for the next few hours?
4. How much do I eat now in order to make sure I have a good appetite for my next meal? (I know I will enjoy my meal so much more if I eat it with a good appetite.)

Most of us discount how foods make us feel over time; instead, we eat to feel good in the moment, only to suffer the painful consequences afterward. If only the pain of overeating or eating foods that are difficult to digest happened in the moment, a lot fewer people would overeat! Unfortunately, the pain of stuffing ourselves occurs later, after we walk away from the table or the fast-food counter and notice how uncomfortable our body feels. How long does the pain last? It depends on what you eat, but it might last for thirty minutes to an hour if you've overeaten a small amount, or for hours or even days if you've had a real blowout. So you trade a few minutes of pleasure for hours of pain.

Think about it: how long does it take to consume a cookie or a candy bar? A minute? Maybe two. How long does it take you to eat a whole meal? Probably less time than you think. I've read studies that say that most Americans plow through dinner in seven minutes or less. Seven minutes! Time yourself next time, and see how long your actual eating time is. We finish quickly, yet we may feel the negative effects in our body for an hour or two afterward. That's a bad deal, wouldn't you agree? It reminds me of credit card debt. We experience the short-lived pleasure of buying things but months or years of pain trying to pay off the balance at high interest rates.

Food for Thought

If you're someone who says, "I eat what I eat because I just love to eat," it suggests to me that you are exaggerating the pleasure of the experience of eating for the minute or two you are eating but discounting the discomfort and the displeasure over the next hour or two that the food will negatively affect your body. What would it be like if you shrank the momentary experience of eating down to the small experience it is and expanded the pleasure of eating in harmony with your body? The instant gratification might look like a small dot in a big blue sky. What if that's the same sky in which your dreams will take flight?

A naturally slim and healthy person makes the best investment in her body. She eats in a way that makes her feel better for longer.

Imagine that—an eating strategy that brings you more pleasure from food than what you're getting now. To "install" the naturally slim and healthful eating strategy in your subconscious mind, dig into the exercise below, adapted from the pioneering work of Connirae Andreas in her book *Heart of the Mind.* I use the word "install" because by walking through the steps below and rehearsing them as recommended, you will actually be installing this strategy in your subconscious, giving your mind a pattern to follow that already feels familiar. Remember that the subconscious mind doesn't know the difference between something vividly imagined and what's actually happened in real life. So settle down and dig in!

Dig In: The Naturally Slim and Healthful Eating Strategy

Let's say it's close to noon and your office mates are beginning to pack up and head out for lunch. Before jumping up and automatically heading out the door with the rest of the gang, you take a brief moment to assess your hunger. You place your hands on your stomach (remember: the stomach is just below the rib cage, above the belly), and you ask yourself, "How does my stomach feel right now?" Tilt your head down, close your eyes, and notice the physical feeling in your stomach. You determine that you're at about 1 on the hunger scale and heading out to lunch is a good idea because you're quite hungry.

Once you determine that you're truly physically hungry, ask yourself, "What would feel good in my stomach over time?" Take a mental inventory of the foods and the portion size that will feel good in your stomach. Notice, I said what will feel good *over time*, not what will taste good in the moment. (Just to be clear, taste is very important. Food should always be enjoyable, and it should also feel good in your body for as long as possible. You want and deserve both.)

Put your hands on your stomach, and imagine tasting the food you're thinking of eating. Imagine the sensation of chewing and swallowing the food and the food entering your stomach. How does the food feel in your stomach over time? Imagine it in your stomach over an hour, two hours, and then three hours. What's that like? Face it: the food you eat will probably be with you, in active digestion, for at least an hour or more, depending on what and how much you eat. It's not in your mouth for very long, but it's in your body for quite some time. Do you like how it sits with you over time? Check in and find out. Does it make you feel light, energized, or sluggish? Does it give you an even amount of energy to keep going or a quick boost followed by a crash? How does eating it affect your enjoyment of the next meal? How does it affect the rest of your afternoon or evening? Does it make you more alert as you go through your day or slow you down? Finally, ask yourself, "Do I like it? Overall, do I like the way this food makes me feel physically?"

If you like how the food you've imagined eating makes you feel over time, save it as your best option so far. If you don't like how the food will sit with you, consider another eating option and go back through the steps. Repeat the process until you've determined the food that will give you the most satisfaction over the longest period of time. Once you've identified the food that will make you feel the best for the longest time, congratulate yourself, because you've just chosen to maximize both your pleasure and your enjoyment!

It may not be easy to remember to ask yourself all these questions each time you think about eating, but because the steps are written in the sensory-based language of the subconscious, they tend to sink in quickly.

I often have my clients literally walk through a series of numbered steps to install the naturally slim and healthful eating strategy in their minds, and you might find this approach helpful, too. Make seven cards as labeled below, place them on the floor, and step through them a few times until your brain locks the steps into place.

1. Cue
Something makes you think of food (e.g., seeing it, the time of day, others are eating).

2. Feel
Ask yourself, "How does my stomach feel now?"

3. Hear
Ask yourself, "What would feel good in my stomach *over the next couple hours and beyond?*"

4. See
Imagine a portion of food.

5. Feel
As you consider eating it, taste it, feel it sliding into your stomach, and feel it in your stomach *over time.* Do you like it?

6. Compare
Compare this feeling to the best option so far.

7. Save or Discard
Save the image as the best option, or mentally grab the image and throw it away.

With a little practice, you will notice yourself going through these steps almost automatically whenever you think about eating. Also, as you pay more and more attention to the eating experience and how different foods and how much of them affect you over time, you will develop an internal inventory of what foods satisfy you the most under what conditions. Soon enough, you'll find that you instinctively choose foods that give you the biggest bang for your buck, and that is exactly what I mean when I say that the Full-Filled program will change your cravings. Eventually, and maybe sooner than you think, you will start to crave the foods that are the most nourishing and that physically satisfy you for a longer period of time. Perhaps you will have a sudden urge for some dark leafy greens or crave some brown rice or fresh walnuts. That's your body's way of telling you what nutrients it needs and when it needs them.

Someone Who Tried This Before You

Susan is a professional woman in her forties with neat brown hair and a sincere heart under a slightly nervous demeanor. She had been up and down the scale for much of her life, had gone for years at a time being slim, but had always gained the weight back, and then some. A couple years before we met, her mother had become ill and needed Susan's attention. With the strain of frequent visits to care for her mother and her eventual death, she found herself using food for comfort. Self-care went out the window, and her exercise regimen became nonexistent. She gained 45 pounds. After about eighteen months of suffering and realizing she had reached her highest weight ever, she knew it was time for a change. She started by participating in a weight loss program that involved a mind-body approach but found it involved so much work and attention that she couldn't keep up with it. Eventually she came to see me.

By that time she was so leery of weight loss programs and so drained from her mother's death that all she wanted at first was to rediscover her motivation to lose weight. After clearing issues of worthiness and coming to understand the essential value of self-care, she found herself ready and eager to shift her eating behavior and lose weight. I walked her through the naturally slim and healthful eating strategy, and, shortly thereafter, she surprised herself.

Whereas lunch typically involved something heavy, she started to prefer lighter fare. She had had a habit of visiting the vending machine in the afternoons and soon realized that she was craving whole fruit instead because she didn't want to feel heavy for the rest of the day. She also wanted to look forward to enjoying a healthful evening meal on an empty stomach. These small, healthful choices started a beautiful new cycle of eating for Susan. The healthful, satisfying evening meal helped her sleep better at night, which gave her energy for an invigorating morning walk. After just six weeks of practice, her clothes started getting looser and her new norm became ease around healthful eating.

About the naturally slim and healthful eating strategy, another client of mine once said, "You know, I just want to have my treats, and if I follow this strategy, I'm worried that I'll never be able to have treats again." I said, "No, no, no, this plan is not about denying you your treats. It's about eating in such a way that you set yourself up to feel better longer. That's it." Remember, becoming slim and healthy is not an act of omission. Rather, on a daily basis, you will add foods to your diet that make you feel good. Now, you may find that, in fact, healthful food really does that, much more than unhealthful foods laden with caffeine, sugar, salt, and artificial additives, which tend to give you a quick spike of satisfaction followed by a crash. Everything that those foods give you in a short amount of time, they take away twofold or more in the immediate hours afterward. And those foods can have negative effects on you for days, weeks, and months after you've eaten them. Did you know that if you're overweight, you're carrying around the excess junk food you ate a year ago? Yuck! So the goal of the naturally slim and healthful eating strategy is to eat the foods that make you feel the best over time. Eventually, you just may find that your go-to "treat" doesn't do that for you.

That is exactly what my client discovered. After walking through the naturally slim and healthful eating strategy a few times, she was astounded to discover that when she thought about having a treat, the first things that popped into her mind were foods such as hard-boiled eggs and bananas. When I asked her, "What changed?" she answered, "You know, I'd rather snack on an egg or a banana in the afternoon when I'm hungry, because those are the kinds of foods that will put me in the exact right hunger spot so I can really enjoy dinner with my family."

Food for Thought

If you say to yourself, "I deserve a treat," as you walk past the office goodies, stop and take a minute to think about what you qualify as a treat. Is a "treat" something that puts extra calories, saturated fat, cholesterol, and processed substances into your body? Is that really what you deserve? Don't you deserve to feel better than that? Don't you deserve to feel good in your body all afternoon and really enjoy your next meal? Reconsider what a real treat is.

As you establish a habit of checking in with your hunger and listening to your body's natural cues, will you always make the best food choices? More than likely, no. From time to time you'll eat something that turns out to be richer and heavier than you expected. No worries! This is not a problem, because when you do choose foods that don't make you feel good over time, you will simply self-correct. The slim and healthful eating strategy has self-correction built right into it.

So if you eat something heavy such as a double cheeseburger and fries that leaves you feeling sluggish and run down, relax. Practice the Re-Do. Go back in time and re-do the experience as you would have liked it to go, either making a different choice or stopping eating sooner. Replace the urge to overdo it with a feeling of relaxed ease, and enjoy the lasting satisfaction that follows. Then, the next time you're hungry and you check in with your body about what foods will make you feel the best over time, you probably won't imagine a double cheeseburger, will you? Instead, you'll likely imagine and choose lighter foods that sit better with you and are therefore more pleasurable to eat.

That's what we're after here: maximizing your pleasure over time. Does that sound like hard work? Does that sound like deprivation? I don't think so. Eating for pleasure is the secret to becoming naturally slim and healthy. It's true: you get to choose to eat foods that make you feel fantastic and lose weight in the process. What a deal!

 Food for Thought

So much of the diet and weight loss industry promotes the message that you're going to have to struggle, sacrifice, deprive yourself, and have tremendous discipline in order to be slim and healthy. That's just not the case. The great surprise about the naturally slim and healthful eating strategy is that it not only is easier than all that but will actually bring you much more pleasure from food than you get now. How great is that?

Throughout the weeks ahead, the only thing I want you to deprive yourself of is overeating. Notice I said *overeating*, not eating. I want you to eat, and I want you to enjoy every bite that you put into your mouth. What I do want you to lose is the uncomfortable feelings of never feeling hungry or feeling too full. Those are both low-enjoyment experiences. High-enjoyment eating is when you arrive at a meal hungry and you taste all the flavor of what's on your plate, setting your fork down when you're just satisfied and arriving at your next meal ready to enjoy your food all over again. When you focus on maximizing your enjoyment and pleasure and letting go of eating experiences that make you feel bad, you will discover true satisfaction. It's a win-win!

Someone Who Tried This Before You

Ginger was at the airport waiting for her flight to board when she suddenly got a craving for a coffee and a chocolate chip cookie. She decided to give in to her craving, and the first two bites of the chocolate chip cookie were heavenly. She told me that they satisfied her craving perfectly. Yet after bite two, the taste of the cookie started to lose its pizzazz. Not wanting to waste a perfectly good cookie, she finished it anyway and then proceeded to feel physically bad for hours afterward. As we spoke about it in our session, she said, "I shouldn't have bought the cookie. I should have chosen differently. If only I hadn't eaten the whole thing." She was really beating herself up over it.

"Now, hold on," I said. "There's two ways to work with this." First I encouraged her to let go of the guilt. "You're imperfect. You overate. Big deal. Now you have an opportunity to learn from this experience." Then I suggested that she create two separate Re-Dos: one where she stopped after two bites, maximized her enjoyment of the experience, and avoided hours of physical discomfort, and the other, where she passed on the cookie altogether and chose a more healthful option, such as fruit, that would likely have left her feeling better over time.

I didn't scold her for eating a cookie. I didn't suggest she never eat cookies again. As far as I'm concerned, all foods are allowed. Eat what you love to eat. Just be honest about how they make your body feel. I simply suggested that in her Re-Do she let go, or deprive herself, of bites five, six, and seven because those were the bites of the cookie that had led to her feeling awful. "Eat the cookie if you like," I told her. "Just stop eating it when the enjoyment fizzles."

I think I've made this point loud and clear, but I'll say it again anyway: the point of the Full-Filled program is not to turn you into the perfect eater. Remember, a black-and-white, all-or-nothing approach won't get you anywhere except higher up on the scale. Also, perfection doesn't promote growth, nor is it really achievable. Instead of seeking perfection, remind yourself that you are on a path of continuous improvement where sometimes you'll choose cookies and wish you hadn't. No biggie! Naturally slim and healthy people sometimes overeat, as do I. It's going to happen. And when it does—when you eat past the point of enjoying your food—you will simply self-correct and chalk it up to a learning experience. You're on a journey marked by opportunities to improve and grow. Just like a baby learning to walk, you, too, will fall down and get right back up—a little dinged but open to the adventure of exploring life and standing tall.

Reeducate Your Palate

It's human nature to want what we can't have, so if we forbid ourselves to have something, we will likely increase our desire for it. For that reason, I don't like to put a cease and desist order on any foods in your pantry. However, I think it's important that you understand what foods have the longest-term payoff. In this section, I'll discuss what foods are better to eat, not in the context of what you should or shouldn't eat but rather in the context of what foods will be more enjoyable to you over time and therefore make it easier for you to be slim, fit, and healthy for a lifetime. Take it from me, you want your weight-release journey to be easy, because if it's not, when push comes to shove, any difficult step will be the first to go.

Before we get started, I should mention that I'm not a nutritionist or a scientist, but I do know a lot about food because I was obsessed with it for many years. I studied everything I could find on the subject, as have many of my clients, who have an encyclopedic knowledge of nutrition. You probably know a lot about food, too.

The Full-Filled program is all about enjoyable, easy weight release, so what do you imagine are the foods that will make it easier for you to be naturally slim and healthy for a lifetime? Maybe the best approach is to first identify the foods that *won't* make it easy. To do that, let's take a quick look at the creation of food science.

In the 1960s, food scientists went to work to create foods that would be cheap to produce, wouldn't spoil, and would have lengthy shelf lives. While they were at it, they also sought to design foods that tasted so good that we'd make a habit of eating a lot of them, over and over again. It was a tall order, but they did it. Cheaply produced processed foods—chock-full of hidden ingredients such as petroleum and industrial solvents—started appearing on grocery store shelves in the 1970s, and more than four decades later, we're still gobbling them up. Those foods have been engineered in such a way that they outlive fresh foods by months, sometimes years, and scream "Flavor!" to our taste buds.

Think about it—you can't eat just one Dorito, can you? It's impossible, and that's because they've been engineered to mess with our true hunger signals and enhance our cravings. Make no mistake, they're specifically designed to make us want to eat more and more of them. Unfortunately, they're not very good for our bodies. Because our bodies did not evolve eating foods full of chemical flavorings and consistency enhancers, they are poorly equipped to deal with them. Our bodies expect nutrition, and they just don't get it when we eat processed foods.

The first step in creating a food plan that will make it easier for you to become naturally slim and healthy is to cut out foods that contain ingredients that the body finds particularly confusing. My first rule of thumb is to cut back on, or stop eating altogether, foods that contain "unpronounceables"—ingredients you can't pronounce, such as monoglycerides and diglycerides. If you can't pronounce it, your body probably doesn't know what to do with it, which means you probably shouldn't eat it! As a general rule, look for foods with five or fewer ingredients, all of which you can pronounce and identify. In addition to cutting back on foods that contain ingredients you aren't familiar with, I suggest you reduce your intake of foods that contain the following ingredients.

Trans Fats

Trans fats are in many of the packaged foods we eat today, and these fats go into your body and almost never come out. There is no amount of trans fat that is safe for human consumption. The food industry loves trans fats for their shelf stability and for the flaky, crispy quality they give to baked and fried goods, yet our bodies don't know how to process them. Ironically, they were invented as a more healthful replacement to saturated fats, but as it turns out, trans fats are worse for you. If possible, completely remove trans fats in the form of hydrogenated and partially hydrogenated oils from your diet. They do nothing for you other than raise your cholesterol, increase your chance of developing heart disease, and confuse your body. Not a winning combination. Many commercially produced crackers, cookies, and cakes, and many fried foods, such as doughnuts and french fries, contain trans fats. Shortenings and some margarines can be high in trans fats, too. Look for the words "partially hydrogenated vegetable oil." That's just another term for trans fat. While trans fats lurk in many of our foods, many manufacturers are creating substitutes due to increased public demand, yet we still have a long way to go before they disappear from our store shelves completely, so read food labels before you throw anything into your cart (and into your mouth!). *Note:* At this time in the United States, foods can be labeled "Trans Fat–Free" and still contain trace amounts of trans fats.

High-Fructose Corn Syrup

High-fructose corn syrup (HFCS) is a highly refined sweetener developed from corn that is prevalent in the United States and is processed and modified at high temperatures. It's very cheap to manufacture, sweeter than table sugar, and extremely stable on the shelf, so food manufacturers love it. It's in most of the foods on your supermarket shelves, often where you least expect to find it, including in bread, yogurt, granola, energy bars, protein drinks, and even some "natural" products. The big problem with high-fructose corn syrup is that fructose is not metabolized the same way that glucose is metabolized and therefore puts a tremendous strain on the liver when consumed in quantity. Though there is some controversy over how bad it is, I've read research that suggests that when we eat foods containing high-fructose corn syrup, our body somehow doesn't get the message that we're full—and if we don't know that we're full, we continue to eat! That has been my experience. When I eat foods high in HFCS, I end up hungrier after eating them than before I started.

A lot of research, particularly out of the University of California at Davis, suggests that high-fructose corn syrup is directly linked to the increase of obesity in this country. In reaction to all the negative press, the manufacturers of this ingredient have actually proposed renaming it "corn sugar" to give it a better public image. Either way, it is a highly processed substance, it's very sweet, and it seems perfectly evident to me, and I hope it does to you, too, that eating it will not make becoming naturally slim and healthy any easier. What *will* make your life easier is eliminating it from your diet or dramatically reducing your consumption of it. If you decide to eliminate it from your diet completely, expect the transition to be a little rocky as you search for foods to replace those that contain high-fructose corn syrup, but once you get into the habit of choosing alternatives, you will quickly find it easy.

Food for Thought

By moving away from processed foods and towards more organically grown foods that are free of hormones and pesticides, you will reawaken your taste buds to the subtleties of natural nutrition. When you eat natural, healthful foods, you can more easily determine when your body is truly physically hungry. Replacing your intake of processed foods with natural foods will therefore make weight release easier. The transition may be a little bit difficult as you create a list of go-to foods and recipes, but once you get into the habit of buying more healthful, natural foods, you will find it easy to sustain.

Sugar

Sugar consumption in the United States has skyrocketed in the last fifty years. The USDA estimates that every American eats an average of ninety pounds of added sugar per year. (That number excludes naturally occurring sugars found in fruits and vegetables.) We all know that moderation is healthful, and this quantity of sugar is anything but. Plus, this is an average across the entire population, so if you have a sweet tooth, you're likely consuming a great deal more. In fact, you're probably unaware of how much sugar you're consuming because it's hidden in so many foods. Would you believe that sugar is often added to basic table salt? It may sound ridiculous, but it's true.

One of the reasons there's so much added sugar in our foods today is that over the years our taste buds have adapted to a sweeter diet and now are used to it. Because as a culture we've gotten so used to added sugar in a wide variety of our foods, it takes a lot of sweetener to fully satisfy our taste buds. As the years go by, we have craved sweeter and sweeter foods, so food manufacturers continue to produce them to satisfy the demand. (Plus, they make a lot of money by doing so.)

There are a number of reasons why eating this much sugar is not good for us. When we eat sugar in any of its many forms, it causes a surge in blood sugar that triggers our bodies to release insulin. Insulin is the hormone that allows our bodies to regulate and control our blood sugar levels and bring them back down into a safe range. When we eat a lot of sugar, the pancreas excretes a tremendous amount of insulin very quickly, and this insulin surge often causes our blood sugar to drop too fast—this is when we experience a "sugar crash." Because sugar is meant to be metabolized slowly, when we eat an overabundance of it, our pancreas gets a workout. Unfortunately, the pancreas wasn't designed for this level of work, so when we repeatedly slam it with sugary foods, it gets worn out and damaged. In addition, our bodies become desensitized to insulin, meaning we need more and more of it to metabolize the sugar in our bodies. In cases when the pancreas finally cries "Uncle!" because it can't keep up with the demand for insulin, we suffer from diabetes (too little insulin in the blood).

As if that weren't bad enough, sugar also puts a strain on the liver. When we eat too much too often, the liver also cries "Uncle!" and stores it as fat. A fatty liver is an unhappy liver and one that doesn't work very well. In short, too much sugar causes a classic overuse syndrome called "metabolic syndrome," which puts you at high risk of developing obesity and type 2 diabetes. Mounting evidence suggests that sugar also puts you at a much higher risk of developing heart disease and cancer. These are the big four health epidemics of our time, and it looks as though they're all related to our increased consumption of sugar.

Does this mean you need to stop eating sugar altogether? Whether or not you eat sugar is a call you'll have to make for yourself, but consider that life may be easier if you remove it from your diet. I didn't think I could do it, but when I was in Overeaters Anonymous, I quit cold turkey and successfully abstained from consuming sugar for sixteen years! It takes the body about three days to eliminate a substance from the system, so if you're addicted to sugar or there is a lot of sugar in your diet—and I speak from experience here—give yourself about three days to get off it. When I did so, I actually had headaches and shakes from the withdrawal, but eventually those effects subsided, along with my cravings for sweets. I actually don't recommend quitting cold turkey as I did. It feels awful and feeds into the all-or-nothing mind-set. Instead, I recommend reducing your intake gradually and substituting natural foods, such as delicious, juicy fresh fruit. You'll find that by reducing your sugar intake by just 50 percent, you'll likely be able to avoid the blood sugar highs and lows that accompany a diet high in sugar, and you will have fewer cravings for the sweet stuff overall.

I did eventually reintroduce some sugar into my diet, but not much. Today, honey, agave nectar, and maple syrup are the preferred sweeteners in my house, but if I'm at a dinner party and there's a particularly good-looking dessert, I may decide to indulge. I always make a conscious choice about eating sweets, though, because I know that they will likely cause a blood sugar crash a few hours afterward and create a sweet craving in me the very next day. That craving can be a drag to deal with, so either I'll plan to be on alert to the craving so I can pass on the urge or I'll decide that eating dessert isn't worth it. If I know I'm going to suffer for eating something, it quickly becomes less appealing, and that makes it very easy to pass up. What if every time you thought about eating sweets, you instantly felt a bit of the uncomfortable and irritable sugar crash to come? Would that alter your decision to buy that candy bar in the vending machine? I bet it would. Once you become hyperaware of how the food you're putting into your mouth will feel in your body over time, your cravings will change. You will start to crave foods that make your life less complicated, easier, and more enjoyable.

Artificial Sweeteners

I used to be a diet soda junkie. I drank it every day, and for a while I even had it at breakfast! I thought, "A hit of caffeine and no calories—what could be better?" Real food, that's what! Paris Hilton summed it up best when she so diplomatically said, "Diet soda is for fat people." Research proves her statement to be right. In one study, lab rats were divided into two groups; one group was given sugar, and the other was given a combination of sugar and artificial sweeteners.

After ten days, both groups were given a supply of unadulterated rat food. The group of rats that had been feasting on artificial sweeteners for ten days ended up eating three times the amount of food as the all-sugar group! Researchers speculate that artificial sweeteners, including aspartame, sucralose, neotame, acesulfame potassium, and saccharin, among others, interfere with our body's ability to judge the energy content, or calories, in our food. Like high-fructose corn syrup, artificial sweeteners confuse our natural hunger signals.

Barbara Rolls, a researcher at Pennsylvania State University, says, "As foods get more and more dissociated from our traditional history with foods, it's going to be harder and harder for us to regulate how much to eat." Why not make your life easier and move away from "unpronounceables" and ingredients that are difficult for your body to digest and towards food that is closer to its natural state? You'll feel better, you'll look better, and add to that the fact that your body burns more calories when digesting whole foods than when digesting processed foods. That's a pretty good trade-off, if you ask me.

The Secret of Changing What You Crave

In one of the first weight-release group classes I taught at a big high-tech company near San Francisco, I decided to conduct a blind taste test. I scoured local supermarkets for foods with processed and organic equivalents. I carefully set up the blind tasting and had group members rate which foods they preferred on slips of paper. I was looking forward to the minimally processed organic foods winning the taste test and proving my point that natural is better. Well, you can probably guess what happened: the processed foods won hands down. Most everyone preferred them to their organic equivalents. Boy, was I embarrassed.

The good news is that I learned a huge lesson from that class (remember, our mistakes are our teachers!). I realized that in order to prefer healthful foods, we have to reeducate our palates. Foods containing excessive salt, fat, sugar, and flavor enhancers scream "Flavor!" at our taste buds, which have become very lazy. To prefer natural foods, we have to reacquire a taste for subtlety. After I started removing processed foods from my diet, it took some time for my palate to relearn the subtle textures and flavors of natural food. This will probably be true for you, too. As you move away from processed foods and towards healthful, natural whole food alternatives, be sure to slow down and take time to notice and savor their subtle, complex flavors. Many of my clients have discovered that after they gave up their high-sugar and high-salt diets for as little as a few days, they began to taste things differently. As soon as you cut down on the amount of processed foods in your diet, you will reawaken your palate and be able to taste the true flavors of good, healthful food. I think you'll be surprised at how delicious natural foods can be. Imagine organic sprouted grain bread holding more enjoyment than a Dorito!

Someone Who Tried This Before You

Rebecca, one of the many binge eaters I have worked with, started off a visit with me by saying, "You know, I'm not binge eating anymore, but I'm still eating junk food. I should only eat healthy food all the time."

I said to her, "That's interesting. You're not bingeing, which is terrific, but you're still eating junk food."

She said, "Yeah, it's terrible, isn't it?"

I said, "No, it's great. Congratulations! If you can eat junk food and stop before you go too far, imagine how much easier it will be to eat healthy, natural foods in moderation. We know that your change is really stable because you can eat junk food and still eat responsibly and moderately. Not a lot of people can do that, so take it as a sign of how stable your progress is." After that she brought a much more relaxed attitude to her eating and started to notice that she actually enjoyed healthful food more, so she started to eat it more often and her progress was more stable than before.

♥

Claire was a real on-or-off person; either she was highly restrictive and disciplined with her eating, or she ate everything and anything in sight. She began practicing the Full-Filled program and eventually came to the conclusion that restriction was not benefiting her. She told herself, "I've had enough of all this control! I am not going to restrict myself. I'm going to give myself full permission to go out and have incredibly indulgent food from one of my favorite restaurants in town, and I'm going to really enjoy it. I'll take my time and savor every bite." She loved greasy fried food yet never ate it, so she went to a pub that was famous for fish-and-chips and gave herself the green light to eat every last bite, and guess what? After all the years she'd been restricting herself, telling herself that greasy fried food such as fish-and-chips was bad even though it tasted so good, she discovered that she really didn't like it that much. How about that?

After that discovery, she started going down her list of "forbidden foods," giving herself full permission to eat them. She realized that she really didn't have a taste for many of the foods on her list. She'd created the illusion that she loved them only because she couldn't have them. As she became more and more in tune with her body, she discovered that there were actually more healthful foods that she enjoyed a lot more, especially because they made her feel so much better in her body for so much longer.

To begin the process of reeducating your palate to enjoy healthful, natural foods, I invite you to cut down on the amount of processed foods that you eat by 25 percent and then 50 percent, so that over time you improve the quality of the foods you eat significantly.

Replace refined, processed foods with fresh produce (fruits and vegetables that are organically grown and free from hormones and pesticides), complex carbohydrates, lean protein, and natural fats.

Making the shift from what you're currently eating to a diet rich in natural foods may take some up-front work. I encourage you to make the investment. It's well worth it. Plus, I think you'll find that once you get organized and get into a habit of buying and preparing healthful foods, it will no longer seem like work. Rather, eating in a more healthful way will become easy and intuitive. Eating healthfully feels like hard work only if you're feeling deprived. Remember, the only thing I want you to deprive yourself of on the Full-Filled program is eating foods and portions of foods that make you feel bad. The reason to eat healthful food is to maximize your pleasure and enjoyment while nurturing your body. And that's the only reason to eat!

As you come to prefer natural, healthful foods, you may want to set your intent to align your appetite with a slim and healthy body. Allow this mindful meditation to help you reset your hunger levels to slim, while your body uses the handy stored energy it's been carrying around to meet more of your daily energy needs.

Mindful Meditation: Align Your Appetite with Slim and Healthy

You may have already begun to feel less like a slave to your cravings and more like the master of your pleasure and enjoyment. The tools you have been using have given you the freedom to do this. Take a moment now to drop inside and thank your body for all it does for you. You know how hard it's been working to digest and store all the extra food you've been eating. You can now let it know that it's time for a break. Your body can now use the stored energy that's already there in the form of fat to fuel part of your daily energy needs. There's a source of energy right in your body, ready to be used and released. Set your intent to utilize some of that stored excess energy each day as you reach a slim and healthy weight.

Produce

Fresh produce is always a great choice. As Michael Pollan, author of *The Omnivore's Dilemma* and *In Defense of Food*, advocates, "Eat food. Not too much. Mostly plants." Naturally packed with nutrients, water, and fiber, fruits and vegetables are satisfying and nutritious, and of course the natural fiber in them aids with digestion and elimination. I recommend that you make sure your lunch and dinner both include a large dose of veggies, such as a salad or a vegetable soup, and I recommend fruit with breakfast and as a filling, energy-boosting snack when you get hungry during the day.

Note: When buying produce, I recommend choosing organic whenever possible because organic foods often have a fuller flavor and less pesticide and antibiotic residue, and they're packed full of nutrients. Plus, organic farming is good for the planet. "But buying organic is too costly," you say. A little-known fact: Americans spend a smaller portion of their household income on food than almost any other nation, so although high-quality organic food may seem expensive, it's really a relatively small investment in your health, and eating this way is certainly cheaper than paying expensive medical bills. Plus, when you eat the Full-Filled way, you'll be more satisfied with less food, so savings are built right into your purchases!

Carbohydrates

As far as starches are concerned, complex carbohydrates in the form of whole grains or, even better, sprouted grains are best for your body. Sprouted grain bread is my personal favorite because it retains most of its nutrients. As far as sliced bread goes, the next best thing is whole grain bread. Look for bread products in which the first ingredient is "whole," such as "whole wheat flour." If you are used to white bread, be patient with yourself as you acquire a taste for more healthful varieties, and be patient with your grocery store for its often limited stock of whole grain breads. Last time I checked, I could not find a single loaf in the bread aisle of a traditional grocery store that didn't have high-fructose corn syrup or "unpronounce-bles" in the ingredients. When buying grain-based products, look again for "whole," as in "whole grain brown rice" or "whole wheat flour." White flour and unbleached white flour are processed forms of wheat from which the bran and germ have been removed, along with the nutrients and fiber that go with them. Manufacturers try to replace those nutrients by fortifying their products with vitamins, but they don't restore everything that's lost. As an added bonus, the body uses more energy digesting whole grains than it does in digesting processed flours, so you actually burn more calories while eating them!

Protein

Protein is great because it lasts a long while in our stomachs, meaning it has a long-term payoff. Lean proteins such as sustainably raised chicken, turkey, and seafood are always excellent choices. If you have a taste for fattier proteins such as beef and lamb, I recommend that you eat them extra slowly and chew them thoroughly to aid with digestion. Eating slowly helps your body recognize how filling those richer meats are before you eat too much.

Note: Simple carbohydrates, complex carbohydrates, proteins, and fats digest at different rates. The more slowly a substance digests, the longer it will take for your stomach to notice that it's full, especially if you haven't trained yourself to pay attention. Protein is slow to digest, which is why, when I eat it, I take small bites, eat it slowly, and savor it, giving my stomach time to notice how filling protein is. To round out my meal, I always pair protein with vegetables because of their high water and fiber content. Starting with a filling vegetable dish, such as a salad or light soup, will help you feel full before you dig into richer foods.

Food for Thought

Eat with intention. Begin your meal with gratitude for the food you are about to enjoy and perhaps even for all the people involved in bringing that food to your table—the farmers, truckers, distributors, and grocers. Also, take a moment to visually appreciate your food. Are there vibrant colors and appealing textures? Now enjoy your food with an intention to nurture and nourish your slim and healthy self. Do this with whatever goes into your body. Commit to making "intentful eating" a practice this week, and see what happens.

Fats

Fats last even longer than proteins, and though you should avoid trans fats completely, natural fats such as those found in avocados, nuts, and many oils are fantastic. They have a high nutritional value, and they make you feel satisfied for longer.

Flaxseed oil is the king of oils because of its high omega-3 essential fatty acid (EFA) content. Flaxseed promotes healthy skin, strong hair and nails, optimum brain function, and good elimination. What's not to like? Flaxseed oil is sold in opaque containers to protect it from degrading exposure to light and should be kept cold. I often use it as a salad dressing, mixed with balsamic vinegar. It's also sold as a nutritional supplement. Keep it in the refrigerator.

Though natural oils are great for you, I must say a word here about butter that almost no one agrees with me on, except perhaps the French, who are famous for their butter croissants and rich meat dishes and who have better heart health than we do in the United States. I have long thought that because human beings evolved eating animal fats from the time we were hunter-gatherers, saturated fat can't possibly be as dangerous for us as we've been led to believe. My personal favorite saturated fat is butter. There's no way that butter-like substances, with their colorings and additives, are better for us than real butter. They certainly don't taste better! Because I eat for both health and enjoyment, a bit of real butter is a tasty delight I savor and adore. I'm not recommending that you melt a stick of it in every dish you prepare, but I do think that in small amounts butter is perfectly acceptable and thoroughly appreciated; it can increase your enjoyment of your food.

Finally, nuts are extremely nutritious, especially when they are fresh. Because they contain a lot of oil, they also spoil easily, especially when exposed to light and heat. The shell naturally protects the delicate oil from light and keeps them moist and delicious. Yet these days, it's pretty darn hard to find nuts still in their shells, which is too bad because the shell makes them harder to work for, making us appreciate each rich morsel. Nuts are a high-calorie-density food, so remember that a little goes a long way, and eat them slowly and with a big dollop of appreciation.

Food for Thought

The only lasting reason to prefer healthful food, healthful exercise, and a healthful lifestyle is that they all make you feel great. Eating and behaving in a way that makes you feel fantastic communicates to your subconscious mind that you are worthy of great self-care, the surefire way to stay slim and healthy for life.

Probiotics

Probiotics are helpful bacteria that protect the body from harmful bacteria and encourage the growth of healthful bacteria in the body. Probiotics are good for the gut. Found in foods such as yogurt, kefir, fresh pickles, and live sauerkraut, probiotics do wonders for gut health, facilitate good digestion, and are amazing immunity boosters. Though they have been stripped from processed foods, we need them more than ever because of our increased exposure to antibiotics, either in medicines or by consuming animals that have been raised on them. A few years ago, I had pneumonia, and it really weakened my immune system. Even after I got back on my feet, it seemed I caught every bug that passed my way. My friend Gina Orlando suggested that I include some high-quality probiotics in my diet, and since I started consuming them regularly, I have fantastic immunity and rarely get sick.

Water

I probably don't need to tell you this, but I'll remind you of something you've heard hundreds of times before: drink water. Drinking lots of clear, fresh water is the best way to satisfy thirst. Many people who struggle with their weight are as out of touch with their thirst as they are with their hunger, so I encourage you to begin paying attention to your level of thirst and hydration and drink accordingly. If you feel run down and crave a quick pick-me-up, instead of grabbing a snack, try drinking a glass of cold water first and then assess how you feel. Often a glass of water is all you need.

Balance your diet with fresh produce, complex carbohydrates, lean protein, probiotics, healthful fats, and water and you'll be golden. By moving away from processed foods and towards foods that have more natural flavor, you will reawaken your taste buds to the delicious rewards of natural nutrition. You will find, too, that your body can better regulate your hunger when you eat unadulterated foods that don't confuse your system's natural signals and create instant cravings. By choosing foods that are closer to their natural state, you give your body the opportunity to reignite its hunger signals, leaving you more satisfied with less food.

Food for Thought

Everything I'm telling you about what foods to eat doesn't matter unless you've done the inside-out part of the weight-release journey. Unless you've identified your objections and resolved your inner conflict, unless you've released your limiting beliefs and replaced them with new, empowering beliefs, what you eat doesn't really matter. I want to be clear about this. It is very easy to latch on to specific foods as the answer to your weight struggle. Food is not the answer. The real answer lies in changing your mind-set about food from the inside out.

That's it! Is that too simple? Were you expecting a more complex eating plan? Well, I hate to disappoint you, but the Full-Filled eating plan is very simple: eat good food that will make your life easier and make you feel better. That's all there is to it, so designate the healthful foods that make you feel the best over the longest amount of time, and personalize a menu plan that fits with your unique tastes and lifestyle.

Most weight loss books want you to follow the exact behaviors and habits of the author writing it. Not me. I want you to customize your eating plan to satisfy your particular body. My body happens to like a diet high in complex carbohydrates, veggies, and good fats. Yours might thrive on a higher-protein diet. The combination of foods that works best for you may not be what works best for someone else.

How will you know what foods and in what combinations are

best for you? By checking in with your body and asking it what it wants and needs. Once you get back in touch with your body's natural cues and track your true hunger, you might notice that your body goes on autopilot, naturally selecting the best foods for itself. Just like a pregnant woman who craves the nutrients she needs (a hunger for pickles, for example, can indicate a need for probiotics), you will discover that your new cravings reflect what your body truly needs to thrive and feel satisfied. How cool is that?

To give you an idea of what dishes make my life easier and more pleasurable, I've included several of my favorite recipes and snacks for you to try at the back of this book.

Structure Provides Freedom and Comfort

I've spent a good deal of time this week lauding the merits of checking in with your body and eating only when you're physically hungry, but I must also say a few words on the value of structure and routine. "Structure and routine?" you ask. "I thought this program was about listening to your body's cues and eating intuitively." It is, but while I help you develop a heightened awareness of what and when your body needs to eat, I also want to give you the structural tools to manage your hunger. Managing your hunger will bring greater freedom to your day-to-day life. Yes, freedom. Within structure there is freedom. It may sound counterintuitive, but it's true.

If you have children or have spent any time around children, you know that they thrive on structure. Take a peek into any preschool classroom, and you'll find a very structured environment in which there's a certain time of day for learning, playing, snacking, and resting. In that structured environment, children thrive because there is a sense of predictability that creates feelings of comfort and security. Notice the words I just used: comfort and security. Aren't these the good feelings that so many overeaters look for from their food? Not only can structure help you manage your eating habits, it can also bring comfort and security to your daily life. Double bonus!

To manage my hunger and calorie intake and also leave me feeling safe and comforted around food, I take a three-pronged approach. One, I eat similar foods from day to day; two, I eat three meals a day; and three, I eat at regular times throughout the day. (See "A Week of Eating" at the end of this chapter for a peek into my daily meal plan and exercise routine.) In a nutshell, I keep my meals fairly basic and my mealtimes very predictable.

Why? Isn't variety the spice of life? Though variety can certainly make life interesting, it can also create a lot of confusion and chaos in your body. It's very common for people who struggle with their weight to fall into a "chaos pattern" where they eat at random times during the day and eat lots of different foods, often swinging between extreme hunger and extreme fullness. Those who allow themselves to get extremely hungry use their extreme hunger as an excuse to eat whatever they can grab, which coincidentally is rarely carrot sticks. I once had a diabetic boyfriend who ate like that. He used to let his blood sugar get so low that he *had* to eat the emergency chocolate bar he kept on him at all times. Yes, you read that right. He carried chocolate as a matter of course. Other "chaos pattern" eaters overeat in great excess to extreme discomfort. I used to know a forensic specialist in San Francisco who told me that occasionally bodies came into the morgue with burst stomachs, the result of overeating to death. Obviously, this is an extreme and horrifying example, but I share it as a cautionary tale.

When your eating schedule is unpredictable and disorganized, you create mayhem in your digestive tract; the stomach doesn't know when to anticipate and digest food, and as a result it's very hard to manage your hunger and maintain or lose weight. If you are someone who eats breakfast at eight o'clock one morning and eleven o'clock the next, it's very important that you get out of that chaos pattern and into a habit of eating breakfast, lunch, and dinner at regularly scheduled times.

Sure, there will be days when your routine shifts to accommodate your kids' school schedule, travel plans, a work meeting that's gone long, or a late-night dinner reservation. But on average you want to create predictability around your meals, if for no other reason than to keep your tummy happy. If you always eat lunch at 12:30, for example, your body knows to begin the digestive process before you even sit down to eat because you will have trained your body to anticipate food at that time. (A growling stomach is often the result of missing your tummy's expected mealtime; it started the digestion process before any food came along.)

Predictable mealtimes allow your metabolism to work optimally for smooth digestion, extracting nutrients and satisfaction for long-term health and happiness. Research into circadian rhythms supports the idea that the body functions better on a regular eating schedule and is more likely to store fat when on an irregular schedule, which prevents the body from establishing a natural rhythm. For those reasons, eat your meals around the same time every day.

I also recommend that you get into the habit, if you're not already there, of eating three meals a day. There are always exceptions to the rule, but most people who are naturally slim and healthy eat three meals a day. Also, if you look at people in nearly every culture—in Spain, France, Argentina, and Japan—you will notice that they traditionally eat three meals a day.

Last, I suggest creating a weekly menu of standard foods and meals that you can easily prepare and enjoy. "How boring!" you cry. Not so fast. Every day I consciously choose to eat delicious foods that make me feel fantastic. To me, this isn't boring—it's liberating! I get to eat my favorite foods every day of the week. How great is that? My breakfast, for example, is usually one of three things: a protein shake, oatmeal with nuts and fresh fruit, or whole grain toast topped with natural peanut butter, cheese, or an egg.

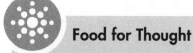

Food for Thought

Human bodies thrive with consistency and regular schedules, so you will want to schedule times when you eat your meals. That way, your body will begin the digestive process in anticipation of the food you're about to eat, and extract as many nutrients as possible from your food. That makes weight release much easier.

Choosing standard meals and mealtimes is like picking out the base model of a car. You will likely "option up" and supplement your meals with a variety of spices, an extra ingredient, or a new preparation, but the basic framework of your meals will remain the same. When you keep your food and mealtimes simple, you create a structured framework that makes your life less chaotic, much easier, and therefore more enjoyable. Plus, research shows that the more novel foods we're exposed to, the more we eat. I believe this is evolutionarily based. Our ancestors' typical diet was extremely repetitive; they ate what was available and in season. When novel foods appeared, they represented novel nutrients that could be important for our health, so we learned to "make room" for them. In our society, where we can have French food for breakfast, Chinese food for lunch, and Italian food for dinner, our cup runneth over with variety, and our waistlines, too. So keep things simple. Set up a standard routine and standard meals. You can get the variety you need by choosing from the various types of produce that are in season and mixing up the grains you eat, for example.

Someone Who Tried This Before You

Emily, a compact woman with curly blond hair, is a dynamo who immediately makes you feel like a close friend. A marketing director at a fast-paced company, she is also the mother of three children, one of whom has special needs. With all she managed in her life, you would never have guessed from meeting her that she suffered from undiagnosed pain and fatigue and often spent days in bed. She was working with a nutrition consultant and weaning herself off a variety of prescription medications in favor of natural supplements when we met. Nevertheless, she still suffered from exhaustion, mood swings, and excess weight.

Emily had what I call a "chaos pattern" of eating. She had no regular mealtimes or standard meals. Every day was a new food adventure, featuring disorienting blood sugar crashes that she would "fix" by consuming more refined sugar. Each meal presented an overwhelming array of choices, as she had no standards, and as a result she often skipped breakfast altogether and struggled through lunch, confused by the multitude of choices available.

Emily was the Rebel personality type. If a diet involved structure and routine, she wanted nothing to do with it, because it reminded her of painful past diets, full of control and restriction. Structure and routine meant having to ignore her body's signals in favor of what the diet of the moment told her she could or couldn't have. Yet she understood that the absence of meal planning was wreaking havoc in her life.

"You're letting your food run your life," I said. "What if I told you that adding some structure to your life would give you freedom?"

She was skeptical, but humbled by her inability to drop the pounds, she conceded. First we released her old negative associations with structure and routine by using the Emotional Freedom Technique. At the urging of her nutritionist, she had already begun eating a natural protein bar for breakfast, and, when she thought about it, she realized that having a standard breakfast had made her mornings much easier. She had never thought about applying the same idea to lunch and snacks.

When we first talked about better options for her snacks (a package of chocolate chip cookies was her favorite go-to), she resisted planning ahead at all. She said, "If I pack some fruit in the morning, what if I don't want it midafternoon? I'll have to eat something I don't want." She was so used to the diet mentality that she hadn't realized that packing a healthful snack, such as fresh fruit or trail mix, would give her an option she hadn't had before. I pointed out that if she had fruit on hand, she could still choose the break room candy bar or she could pass altogether, but now she also had the option of something nourishing and satisfying if she was hungry. When her inner rebel realized that her last-minute approach to eating was actually restricting her and that a little structure and routine could give her the freedom to make better decisions about what and how much to eat, she jumped right on board.

Emily immediately started plotting a new lunch strategy as well. In a follow-up session, she told me how easy it had been to make the adjustment. Since she'd made the shift, she was actually thinking less about food because she no longer worried about getting to a place of starvation and desperation. She was no longer at the mercy of her wild hunger swings. She was free, which is just what her rebel nature always wanted!

Meals: Step by Step and Day by Day

You will begin your day by eating a good, healthful breakfast, preferably with some protein in it (remember: protein has a long-term payoff). Determine how big a breakfast you need to eat by checking in with your stomach and rating your hunger on a scale of 0 to 10. If 0 is famished and 10 is too stuffed to get up off the couch, and if your goal is to lose weight, ideally you want to be at 2 or lower on the hunger scale when you dig into breakfast because you will enjoy your food so much more when you bring a healthy appetite to the table.

If you're someone who doesn't usually eat breakfast because you don't feel hungry in the morning, begin to take note of what you ate the night before. Refer back to your hunger diary. At what time was your last meal, and how much did you eat? Did you finish dinner at a 9 to 10 on the hunger scale? If so, it may account for why you're typically not hungry for breakfast. We often don't realize that how much we ate the night before affects how hungry we are at breakfast. When you stop eating dinner just when you are satisfied and not full, you will arrive at the breakfast table good and hungry.

Until you're able to get into this pattern, if you don't feel hungry when you wake up, simply wait a little while and eat something light, but make sure you eat. Don't skip breakfast; it's the most important meal of the day. It helps wake up your brain and signals to your body that it's time to start burning fuel.

Once you establish that you're hungry for breakfast, eat an amount of food that will leave you satisfied—around 5 to 6 on the hunger scale. Eat until you are satisfied, not full, and then take a break. If you get hungry later, you can always eat more (see the role of snacking in the next section), but until then, put down your fork or spoon and take a moment to appreciate the nourishment you have just given your body and how good it makes your body feel to have just the right amount. Eating to 5 to 6 on the hunger scale will easily get you through the next hours until lunchtime, at which point you'll be good and hungry and ready to eat again. How hungry? Back to a 2 or lower on the hunger scale. Basically, you want to sit down to lunch thinking, "I've worked up a good appetite. I'm really going to enjoy my lunch!"

At lunch, eat as you did at breakfast. Eat an amount of food that will satisfy you and allow you to be nicely hungry at dinner. At dinner, eat enough to feel satisfied but not sluggish or without an appetite the next morning.

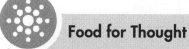

Food for Thought

To release weight, lower your hunger scale numbers from where they were before you started. As you do this, be sure to appreciate how much more you enjoy food when eaten on an empty stomach and take time to savor and appreciate it. Also appreciate how good your body feels for hours after eating, as you have had just the right amount of fuel to energize your day. As a general guideline, go into a meal at 2 or lower on the hunger scale and finish your meal at about 5 or 6. Use these numbers as guidelines only. You alone can determine where on the scale your body feels truly hungry, satiated, and full.

That's it! The rules sound fairly simple, but you're not going to get them right every time. It takes practice, especially if you're at all disconnected from your body's natural cues. No problem. Be patient. It'll take some experimenting and playing around to get it all down. Remember, you can self-correct by checking in with your hunger level whenever you think about food and adjusting your intake accordingly. Over time, you will fall into a very predictable routine that will allow you to manage your hunger, feel safe and comforted around food, and reach your ideal weight.

Dig In: Create a Meal Plan

Create a menu of standard foods and meals that you eat three times a day at regular times. Give yourself options by writing down three standard meals that you enjoy eating for breakfast, lunch, and dinner. Then make a schedule of when you intend to eat each of those meals. Keep a record in your Full-Filled Weight-Release Journal of what and when you ate for the next two weeks of the Full-Filled program to help you establish a regular routine.

The Role of Snacking

Ladies and gentlemen, snacks are part of the Full-Filled program. Starving yourself until your next meal is not necessary, and especially in the early days of your Full-Filled journey, any amount of deprivation is likely to lead you to overeating. Just because you're eating three meals daily doesn't necessarily mean you won't get hungry at other times throughout the day. Say, for example, you've already eaten breakfast and you find yourself starving by 10:30 in the morning. You're already at 2 on the hunger scale, and you know you have a while to go before your midday meal. What should you do? Suffer through it? Go hungry? You've probably been on rigid diets in the past that encourage this. Naturally, I don't.

If you put your hands on your stomach and determine that you are truly hungry—not anxiety or comfort or entertain-myself hungry but physically hungry—you are going to eat. Eat a snack that makes you feel good and tides you over to lunch. It may be something such as an apple or leftover veggies, or if you've been physically active and you're extra hungry, maybe you need a minimeal. Only you can determine what your body needs. Check in with your stomach, and go from there.

The only rule with snacks is that you want to eat just enough so that you arrive at your next meal hungry and maximize your enjoyment. Personally, I love having an afternoon snack, so I purposefully eat a light lunch, stopping at about 4 on my hunger scale, so that I'm good and hungry for my late-afternoon decaf cappuccino and favorite whole grain raisin bun topped with a smear of real butter. I really look forward to taking a break from work to relax and enjoy my snack before returning to the final hours of my workday. In fact, I get rather grumpy if I don't get my afternoon snack break. For that reason, I've built this structure into my day because it keeps my hunger in check and brings me comfort, pleasure, and freedom.

Make It a Ritual

In addition to keeping your metabolism happy and giving you more options and freedom in your life, eating standard meals at regularly scheduled times also allows the eating experience to become a ritual experience. Dictionary.com defines "ritual" as "any practice or pattern of behavior regularly performed in a set manner." I would add that a ritual is something you do on a regular basis that you imbue with meaning and find satisfying. Rituals are comforting, and we often eat for comfort. Personally, I've found that by making my meals a ritual experience, I enjoy them so much more. Plus, I'm less likely to eat past full.

Now, before you start thinking that you need to wear special robes and wave incense around, let me explain what I mean by ritual. Making meals a ritual does not necessarily involve lighting candles, using special linens, or saying a prayer. It can be a very simple act. The only requirement is that you clearly mark the occasion as something different from what you were doing before.

For example, when I eat a snack or a meal, I mark the occasion by sitting down—and not at my desk but somewhere that is clear of work and other distractions—so that I can focus on my food. This simple act communicates to my subconscious mind that I'm transitioning from one activity to another. I also use plates and utensils whenever possible. I want to mark the occasion. Then I take a deep breath and express gratitude for having this time and space in my day and relax, setting an intention to enjoy every bite of my meal. Once I finish eating, I take another deep breath and express gratitude for my meal and for having had the time to appreciate and enjoy it. I've been practicing this meal ritual for years now, and the rare times I don't get it, I feel ripped off! The comfort of my meal sanctuary is not something I want to miss.

Food for Thought

Begin thinking about what you can do in the moment just before you eat to bring a sense of reverence and appreciation to the eating experience. The Full-Filled mind-set is to bring more pleasure into your life, so savor every morsel and allow yourself full appreciation of the sensory experience of eating the food on your plate: the appearance, the taste, the texture, the smell, the way that it feels in your stomach. Appreciate it all.

By making eating a ritual experience where the beginning and end of your meal are clearly defined and imbued with significance as a time for relaxation and renewal, you will find that you eat more mindfully and responsibly, largely because you're more present with your food. Think about it: what often happens when you eat in your car, standing in line, rushing down the street, or sitting at your desk? It's easy to lose track of how much you're eating, isn't it?

When you're not paying attention to the food you're putting into your mouth or how your body feels, you're not really enjoying the experience, and—get this—your body doesn't burn as many calories! When we are on the go and in "stress mode," our metabolism slows down. When we eat when we are calm and relaxed, our metabolism speeds up and we burn more calories. Making your eating experience a ritual not only will bring you comfort and enjoyment, it will directly affect your metabolism and weight.

Mindful Meditation: Ritual Eating

As you think about the food you eat, imagine yourself at your next meal taking the time to set out utensils, a napkin, and a plate or a bowl and to find a place to sit, either alone or with others. Evoke a feeling of appreciation and gratitude and extend it to the food that you're eating. Perhaps it's something that is beautiful and organic and fresh. Even if it's not, take a moment to be grateful for it, to appreciate the fact that it is available to you. Then, as you eat, set the intention that every bit of the food that you eat be utilized by your body to serve its highest good. Imagine your body automatically knowing how best to digest the food in a way that promotes your health and well-being. As your food gently goes down into your body, imagine that anything that it doesn't need is easily released, while it utilizes the nutrients to make you look and feel great.

As you finish your meal, notice how this particular food has made you feel. You may notice that it is a food that you very much enjoyed and want to regularly integrate into your meal plan. Maybe it didn't sit as well with you as you'd hoped. Whatever the case, this awareness will sink down deep inside of you so that the next time you're making a decision about what to eat, you will automatically rely on this feedback to make a better choice.

Now imagine your next meal in just the same way and another meal beyond that. Imagine a whole week's worth of meals. A month's worth of meals. Imagine doing this again and again and again, many times, until the meals all blend together with the overarching intention that everything that you eat be utilized by your body to serve its highest good. Eventually you will start to prefer more healthful foods, the foods that are easiest for your body to work with and make it easiest for your body to be slim, fit, and healthy. Imagine your eating habits aligning with the foods that will bring you optimal nourishment and pleasure. Evoke a sense of appreciation and gratitude for this transformation.

Reliable, Lasting Motivation to Move

This week, we've talked about the importance of tuning in to your body's cues to change your cravings, the foods that will make weight release easy, how to eat for pleasure, and the value of building structure and routine into your lifestyle, yet, as we come to the end of Week 5 of the Full-Filled program, there's one important point we haven't covered: exercise. Believe it or not, everything you've learned about eating for ease and pleasure can be applied to your exercise routine. But before I discuss the striking similarities, let me say a few words about why exercise matters.

In today's world, it's very easy to live a sedentary lifestyle. With modern conveniences and automated appliances and the majority of the workforce spending eight to ten hours a day seated behind desks, a life of limited activity has become the rule rather than the exception. Yet our bodies crave and need physical activity. That's how we're built. From nomadic hunter-gatherers to farmers in the field, the human body has engaged in, adapted to, and thrived on intense physical labor. Today our growing obesity rate reveals a society that's become very comfortable moving less and sitting more, yet our choice to live sedentary lives has led to tremendous suffering. From lack of vitality to excess weight to depression and anxiety, being inactive has inevitable and serious negative consequences, including increased medical bills, lost productivity, and earlier death.

Exercise, on the other hand, has countless benefits. The advantages of exercise reach far beyond the physical, lifting us mentally, emotionally, and spiritually. In fact, studies have found exercise to be at least as effective as some prescription antidepressants. Considering this and given the choice, who wouldn't want to exercise?

What It's Not: Punishment for Overeating

I was not an athletic kid. In fact, in elementary school I was the awkward girl who was the last to be picked for dodgeball or any other team sport in gym class. Nevertheless, as a teen mortified by my expanding waistline and unhealthy eating habits, I discovered exercise was the perfect way for me to atone for my sins and fit in. I'd hit the gym after bingeing on "bad" foods, desperate to work off what I'd just eaten or in anticipation of the next blowout. For me, exercise wasn't about feeling good or being healthy; it was punishment, and it was a way to try to earn some self-worth by transforming my body to meet society's standards.

I've worked with countless clients who approach exercise the same way I used to do—as punishment for overindulging. If they've eaten an excess of 400 calories the night before, they hit the elliptical trainer for an hour or more the morning after for no other reason than to burn off those 400 extra, unwanted calories. I call this the deposit-withdrawal method, and it's not healthful because it's completely guilt-driven and devoid of any pleasure.

Maybe you're wondering why it matters if exercise is guilt-driven if it at least gets you up out of your desk chair and into the gym. Good question. Exercise is a great thing no matter how you get yourself to do it, and guilt-driven exercise is arguably better than no exercise, but guilt-driven exercise increases your stress level, and when your stress level goes up, your metabolic rate goes down, so it's counterproductive. Plus, it's not the most reliable or sustainable practice because it's motivated purely by pain (which is just another word for guilt). Though it's a surefire way to get you revved up and moving, it will keep you revved up for only so long, and that's because motivation based solely on pain wears off because the pain wears off before you've reached your ultimate goal. Pain-based motivation is what gets most people into the gym (especially after the New Year), but it's not a strong enough motivation to keep you coming back on a long-term, consistent basis.

Let me give you an example of what I mean. Imagine that you go to a birthday party and land facefirst in the chocolate cake. The next morning, you feel guilty—and physically awful—so you hit the gym to work off your guilty excess. An hour later, sweaty and fatigued, you feel much better. You leave the gym feeling somewhat redeemed. Whew! What happens the following morning? Do you hit the gym with the same level of intensity and commitment? Probably not—unless, of course, you overate again, but the more likely scenario is that you won't wake up with a food hangover and, given the choice to exercise or not, you choose not to. You reason that you worked out and ate "well" the day before, so why not take a day off? You deserve it, right? Wrong. You deserve to take great care of your body every day so that you consistently feel great physically.

What It Is: Feel-Good "Me" Time

The kind of exercise that's most effective, which is the kind you'll continuously choose to do tomorrow, the next day, and for a lifetime, is motivated by pleasure. Pleasurable exercise—say what? When I lead seminar groups on exercise motivation, I always ask the group, "Whoever hates to exercise, raise your hand." The group is usually split sixty-forty, with the majority of people in the "I hate exercise" category. When I ask them to please tell the rest of us why they hate exercise, they say things such as "Oh, the sweat, I just hate being sweaty" or "I don't have the time" or "It's painful and awkward to put my body in those positions" or "I hate how I look in spandex, and I hate having to face all those mirrors at the gym." Invariably, they emphasize the short-term hassle or pain of exercise and conclude that any positive benefits are too far away.

Conversely, when I ask the group, "Who here loves to exercise?" what do you suppose those people say when I ask them why they enjoy it? With big, bright smiles, they tend to gush about how great exercise makes them feel. That always gets a few snickers, so I ask for clarification, "You love how it makes you feel while you're doing it?" Though some of them say that they like the way they feel while they're doing it, especially if they've found an activity they really enjoy, most of them sing out in protest, "Oh, no! We love how great it feels when we're done."

The majority of people who love exercise emphasize the good feelings they experience after working out and often list specific benefits such as how exercise allows them to be more active with their kids and more present at work and generally gives them more energy to participate in life. It turns out that people who love exercise love it for how pleasurable it feels over time. People who work out in the morning gush over how great they feel throughout the day. Those who exercise in the late afternoon or evening love how much more they enjoy their dinner and the rest of their evening and how well they sleep. Many of them admit that they, too, don't like having to pack a gym bag or change clothes, squeeze into Lycra, and wipe sweat out of their eyes, but for them those concerns take a backseat to the enjoyment of the overall experience. They reason that the initial investment (an hour or so of sweaty, hard work) for a long-term payoff (hours and sometimes days of increased energy, not to mention a fit, toned, healthy body) is worth it. Do you see the similarity between the naturally slim and healthful eating strategy and what I'm describing here?

When you focus on the positive rather than the negative aspects of exercise and approach it as a feel-good activity with immediate and long-term benefits, you'll want to do it more often. Just like choosing more healthful foods that make you feel fantastic for the next several hours after you eat them and make weight release easy to boot, exercise will become something you automatically do to maximize your pleasure and enjoyment of life—today, tomorrow, and into the future.

To rev up your motivation for invigorating exercise, dig into the exercise below.

Dig In: Exercise Pros and Cons

Make a list of the pros and cons of exercise in your Full-Filled Weight-Release Journal. On one side of a blank sheet of paper, write down all of the things that you don't like about exercise; on the other side, write all the things that are really great about exercise (or, if you've never exercised, what great things you've heard or read about exercise). Once you've completed your lists, rewrite them. The second time around, however, write all the things you really don't like about exercise in teeny-tiny small letters, and write what you do like about exercise in beautiful, bold, colorful letters (you may have to borrow some of your kids' crayons or markers for this exercise). As you emphasize the positive and downplay the negative on paper, you will subconsciously do the same in your mind. Your objections will eventually shrink down and fade away, and the benefits will become bigger, brighter, and more appealing!

I exercised like a madwoman all the way through my battle with food addiction (I even worked for a while at a gym because I believed it was the only way I could counteract and control my binge eating), and today I still work out five to six days a week. The difference between how I exercise now and how I exercised then, however, is that today I truly enjoy it. It's not something I have to talk myself into. I really want to do it. In fact, I'm blissfully addicted to it, and the reason for this is that I've transformed exercise from a guilt-driven punishment for overeating into a personal retreat of feel-good "me" time. Because self-care is so important to my overall health and happiness, I've structured my work and family life to accommodate my six-days-a-week exercise routine.

That said, I'm not a machine. I'm human just as you are, and as much as I love to exercise, there are days when I wake up and think it would be nice to linger in bed a little longer than usual, skip my workout, and head straight to the kitchen for a hot, frothy cappuccino and a bowl of warm oatmeal. Certainly no one would notice if I skipped a day. My body would look about the same if I didn't, so in many respects, it's the perfect crime. What stops me? I know that if I skip my morning workout, I won't feel as good later in the day. It's that simple. Exercise makes me feel vital and alive, and I miss those feelings when they're absent. So today, tomorrow, and the day after, I'll drag myself to the closet, pull on my workout gear, and get moving because by doing so I will feel fantastic both immediately and for hours afterward.

I regard my daily exercise routine as a pleasurable, indulgent, and self-serving act because there's no other reason for doing it other than that it makes me feel so darn good. If you've been an exercise hater, I bet you've never thought of exercise like this before. I encourage you to try looking at exercise as something you do as a way to treat yourself exquisitely and take fabulous care of your mind, body, and spirit, because once you do, I promise you will have a totally different experience at the gym, on the trail, in the pool, or on the court. If you're someone who's always hated or dreaded exercise, this may seem hard to believe, but what if I'm right? It's worth a try, isn't it?

If you don't believe you deserve to treat yourself well, if you don't feel worthy of great self-care, it will be a constant struggle for you to do things such as exercise, eat well, and get sufficient rest. If you have this issue, which is actually very common for people who struggle with their weight, how the heck can you address it? You can address your limiting beliefs about worthlessness (which is exactly what avoiding self-care is all about) by using the Emotional Freedom Technique. Create an intention statement and tap on it. Here are a few suggestions:

Even though I don't feel worthy, I still choose to take great care of myself.

Even though I hate getting sweaty (hate dragging myself out of bed, hate workout clothes that make me feel fat), I still choose to enjoy getting physical exercise, and I forgive, love, and accept myself just as I am today.

Go back to the practices introduced in Week 4 of the Full-Filled program and work on releasing your limiting beliefs and replacing them with empowering beliefs about self-care and exercise.

Do What You Love

My body loves cardio, so that's the kind of exercise I do most. Three to four mornings a week I run, ride my bike, or spend an hour on the elliptical machine. (For those of you who resist stationary exercise machines, let me share my secret to making them pleasurable and fun. I used to resist them, too, until I asked someone who enjoyed them how she passed the time. She told me she finds stationary exercise machines meditative and enjoys catching up on reading and podcasts. Brilliant! I was wondering how I could fit meditation into my routine and, voilà, I can just close my eyes on the cardio machine to nowhere and focus on my breath or just let my monkey mind jump to whatever thought it wants to for a while. If I want to feel more engaged with the outside world, I use the time to catch up on my favorite magazines, DVR programs, or podcasts.)

The other two mornings, I start with twenty to thirty minutes of cardio and then focus on weight training and stretching. I also love to dance, so I slip in a heart-pumping dance class whenever I can. Plus, I love to work bonus exercise into my day: walking to shops, riding my bike instead of driving the car, taking the stairs instead of the elevator or escalator.

My exercise routine is fairly predictable but varied enough to keep me interested, and, most important, it works for me. My husband has a routine that consists mainly of yoga. Yoga just doesn't do it for me. Yoga is hugely popular here in San Francisco, where I live, and has many benefits, so I've tried to like it many times, but for whatever reason, I can't get into it. So I accept that and stick with what I enjoy.

As you integrate exercise into your new, active lifestyle, it is essential to figure out how your body likes to move. Let enjoyment be your focus, especially the way being active makes you feel great long after you finish. When you engage in activities you love, you'll want to do them more often. In an effort to discover or rediscover what type of physical activity your body loves to do, dig into the following exercise.

Dig In: Do What You Love

Take a few deep breaths, tune in to that wonderful, miraculous body of yours, and ask it how it likes to move. Let go of what your best friend, your neighbor, or your coworkers do. Forget about the exercises that you've read or heard about that burn the most calories and fat. Instead, focus on calling to mind the activity that really makes your body sing. Take a few moments and ask your body, "What sounds absolutely deliciously delightful to do right now?"

Maybe it's simply going for a walk around the block. Maybe it's taking a hike in nature. It could be taking a bike ride through the countryside or a spin class at a gym. Your body might love yoga, Pilates, or tai chi. It might respond better to traditional weight training or aerobics classes. Maybe it feels best on the basketball court or in the pool. Perhaps you're someone who loves to dance the tango or the two-step.

Once you have your answer, pause for a moment and imagine how great it would be to do the activity regularly. Notice how great you will feel immediately afterward and how feeling that way affects other parts of your day or evening. What are the short-term and long-term benefits of feeling good in your body? Focus on those positive benefits. They will get you moving and keep you moving!

"Doing what you love is easier said than done," you think. Imagining yourself on the dance floor is much easier than finding an available class, signing up for it, and actually showing up. Fair enough, but before you get discouraged and decide to throw in the gym towel, you're going to pause, take a deep breath, and take it one step at a time.

The first step is to think about what it would take to get ready for your workout. What is involved? Signing up for a class? Buying special workout clothes or exercise gear? Making time at the beginning, middle, or end of your day? Putting it on your calendar? Think about what needs to happen to make the activity a reality, and make a list in your weight-release journal. If this step seems too big to accomplish, break it down into smaller steps. You'll know you have the right-size step when you think, "I can do that." For example, if your first step is to hire a trainer and you feel overwhelmed just thinking about it, break it down to a smaller step: search personal trainers in your town or on the Internet or talk to a friend who really likes her trainer.

If you bump into a roadblock such as "I must hire a personal trainer to get myself moving, but they are all too expensive and I can never afford it," try a different approach. Ask yourself, "How else could I learn a good workout routine?" When you ask the right questions, you start to get answers. You could buy or rent an exercise DVD (the library has some for free!). You could look into classes at your local community college. You could check out the YMCA. You could buy a book or recruit a workout buddy. Whatever it is, identify that first small, doable step that will get you moving.

Once you've nailed down the first step, write down the next step in your weight-release journal. Keep going until you've written down all the steps that you can think of in small, doable increments. Again, you'll know the step is the right size if you think, "No problem, I can do that," when you read it. Now attach a date to each actionable step, including a date to start your new physical activity.

As you tackle each of the steps, I want you to be mindful of what you're working for and why. In other words, what's the payoff? If you don't know the answer already (meaning that I haven't successfully drilled it into your head yet), the payoff of each of these small steps is how energized and renewed you're going to feel once you start moving that body of yours. And that's not all. The short-term payoff of exercising has ripple effects that will last for hours, days, weeks, and years to come. You may find it easier to focus on your work, family, and friends. You may sleep more soundly at night. You'll likely find yourself in a much better mood because you're feeling lighter, fitter, and more toned. When you think about how each small step will bring you closer to those rewards, you'll become much more willing to take them.

Someone Who Tried This Before You

Meredith was a very intermittent exerciser; most of the time she didn't exercise at all. She hoped that I could help her boost her motivation to become more physically active. In our first session together, I asked her how she might begin to integrate exercise into her weekly routine. She said that the hours after her demanding day job would be the best time for her to hit the gym. "Although," she admitted, "those are also the hours I feel like I should be tidying up the house, working in the garden, or completing personal projects I've started."

I felt exhausted just listening to her and thought, "Gosh, that's a lot!" I asked, "How would you like to feel in the evenings after work?"

She replied, "Oh! I want to feel excited and up and full of life. But the only thing I'm motivated to do in the evenings is sit on the sofa and snack!"

I asked her, "Well, when do you get your downtime? It seems to me like you're up and ready to go a lot of the time, and if I were in your shoes, I'd really want some quality downtime at the end of the day. No wonder you want to sit on the sofa and eat." I suggested that the positive intent of her inactivity was to give her much-needed downtime.

So that she would no longer turn to snacks on the sofa as a substitute for real rest, Meredith realized that if she carved out fifteen minutes in the morning and ten minutes at the end of the day for quiet meditation (an activity she loved), she would have renewed energy for the evening activity of her choice: exercise, gardening, or personal projects.

Our go-go-go, do-do-do culture is all about getting things done, setting goals, accomplishing them, and checking things off our to-do list, and, for many of us, that's how we value our worth. Sadly, the value of downtime is very low in our culture. It's not part of the good old American work ethic. But we're not machines. In fact, even machines need to be taken offline from time to time for maintenance.

If you, like Meredith, feel unmotivated to exercise, ask yourself, "Am I getting enough quality downtime in my day?" If your answer is no, perhaps the first step in becoming more motivated to exercise is to schedule high-quality downtime into your daily routine. How will you know if it's high quality? When you think about it, you will feel renewed. So there you have it: increase your motivation to exercise by increasing the high-quality downtime in your life.

Create a Schedule

If you read earlier that I work out five to six times a week and thought, "I really hope Renée doesn't expect me to follow her lead," you're right. I don't expect you to go from zero to full tilt overnight—although exercising five to six days a week is certainly a great goal to work up to. What I do recommend is that you put an exercise routine into place that you can consistently commit to. There's that word again: *routine.* Just as with eating healthful foods at regular times, exercise needs to be consistent and predictable in order for it to be easy. If it's not easy, you won't do it. I've found that having a predictable exercise routine allows me to turn my brain off. I don't have to think about when or if I'm going to exercise because I've already put a structure into place that answers those questions for me.

Only you can determine the routine that will fit into your current lifestyle, but I usually challenge new clients who are sedentary to set a goal to work out three times a week. This could be three long walks or three ten-minute bursts of cardio dance moves in your living room. Again, you will make the call. What's most important is that you simply increase your exercise from what you're doing now and create some structure around it so that you continue to do it. If you already exercise, I encourage you to either increase your intensity or add a workout to your existing routine. If what I'm outlining here sounds like too much of a time commitment, let me gently remind you that everyone has the same twenty-four hours in a day. If the president of the United States can make time to break a sweat on the basketball court, you can make time to exercise, too. Saying you don't have time to exercise is code for "My health and happiness are not priorities for me."

Someone Who Tried This Before You

A client of mine named Addison came to me with an exercise "chunk-size" problem. She really wanted to establish an exercise routine but felt that if she couldn't carve out time for hour-long workouts, she shouldn't bother. She belonged to a gym but spent so many hours at the office that she hardly ever made it there.

She told me that a coworker of hers who was also trying to make time for exercise often invited her to take walks at lunch, but she usually declined because "Why bother? A walk doesn't count as a workout. I mean, what's a walk a few blocks around the office at lunchtime compared to a full-blown workout?"

So we talked about changing her perception of exercise so that she'd regard all movement as time well spent. I explained that walking for twenty minutes at lunchtime absolutely counted, especially if she couldn't find time for anything else. Twenty minutes would be great. It would certainly be better than nothing!

It took her a while to come around, but she decided that if twenty minutes a day was all she had, she might as well make the most of it. She set a new goal to exercise three times a week for twenty minutes. It might be ten minutes at lunch and ten minutes on the treadmill after work. It might be getting outside for five minutes of movement four times throughout the day or taking the stairs instead of the elevator. It didn't really matter what she did as long as she did something. It all counted.

Once she started doing this, she discovered how great it made her feel and what a sense of accomplishment it gave her. She began to track her progress, and as she did, she realized, "Wow! Twenty minutes a day does make a difference." From there, her motivation to exercise grew, and before she knew it, she'd increased her twenty-minute workouts from three times a week to four or five times a week. After a short while, she was feeling so good that she rearranged her schedule to fit in a longer workout each week as well.

If you don't currently exercise at all or if you exercise sporadically, getting into a routine will take some time and effort. Don't worry. Be patient with yourself, and consider creating a support system and putting tools into place to help you stay motivated and accountable. For instance, you might:

1. Join a gym and attend group classes.
2. Recruit your weight-release buddies, friends, or neighbors to commit to a similar workout routine and check in with them weekly.

3. Join a walking or running group. Often sporting goods stores or running clubs sponsor them, or ask around at social events if anyone knows of a group.
4. Hire a trainer to set you up and keep you on a regular schedule.
5. Invest in exercise equipment that you keep at home and can pull out in a pinch. (I got a used elliptical trainer that I positioned right near a TV. You can often find great deals on used equipment once you start looking around.)

A Week of Eating

To give you a peek at how I structure my life and how I think about food and exercise, I've included several of my personal weight-release journal entries over the course of a week from the early days of my own Full-Filled transformation.

DAY 1   DAY 2   DAY 3   DAY 4   DAY 5

7:15 A.M. As I awaken, a quick survey of my body—nothing strained, swollen, or torn—reveals that all systems are go for my workout this morning. But first I must put fuel into my body. I eat my standard oatmeal breakfast with a handful of grapes, a dollop of whole milk, live yogurt, and sprinkled walnut pieces.

8:30 A.M. At Golden Gate Park, and the weather is terrific for a run. A balmy 55 degrees. After 4.5 years of chronic fatigue, I'm grateful to be out among the fresh smells of nature in a fit, healthy body that moves.

12:45 P.M. Hungry again after my morning run, I enjoy my usual vegetarian lunch at a local healthful lunch spot that features a small pie of veggies in a whole grain baked crust and a salad. I dab my fork into the tasty Caesar dressing so I can get a bit with every bite, rather than drown the salad in it.

2:30 P.M. I'm on a client call, and my stomach is making noise. I'm booked through until after four, so no time for a snack. I drink a tall, cool glass of water and feel reenergized.

4:30 P.M. Another tall glass of cool water and my favorite whole grain raisin bun, toasted with a light coating of butter on top. More water afterward, and my body sighs contented relief.

7:15 P.M. I'm at about 1 on the hunger scale, so I'm ready for dinner! A few sips of an Italian red wine ease my way into the meal. The wine is an indulgent addition to a Tuesday evening. Tonight I make lasagna with whole wheat lasagna noodles, a couple jars of spaghetti sauce, a can of diced tomatoes, cottage cheese (instead of ricotta), a few sliced zucchini, carrots, onions, and some cannellini beans, topped with Parmesan and Cheddar cheese. Yum.

9:00 P.M. An hour later my stomach reminds me that veggies don't keep it busy very long, so I eat a small bowl of whole grain cereal. I could have eaten more at dinner, but I like to give my stomach a chance to notify my brain of its status. I reason that I can always eat something later if I want, and I often do. This may seem like a roundabout routine, but it's become a fun game to finesse the amount of food that will allow me to sleep well and give me enough energy for my morning workout but not leave me feeling too full or uncomfortable.

DAY 1   **DAY 2**   DAY 3   DAY 4   DAY 5

7:15 A.M. The day starts normally enough. Oatmeal, fruit, and a particularly delightful homemade decaf cappuccino with whole milk, one of my great pleasures in life. I wasn't able to work out this morning, so instead, I hoof it to and from the BART train for a downtown appointment. I love walking for transportation—bonus exercise, beautiful scenery, fresh air, interesting shops and people to look at. Today it was a total of about forty minutes of walking, round-trip, fast-paced, with the added bonus of BART stairs. Yes,

I walk up stairs instead of taking the escalator, no matter how many there are. Why not? It's bonus exercise that lifts the derriere.

12:30 P.M. Thai veggies, tofu, and brown rice. Just right.

2:00 P.M. My stomach is growling, so a whole wheat raisin bun with a light coating of butter and my second decaf cappuccino of the day. Relaxing and renewing, it's a small sanctuary spot in my day.

4:45 P.M. An apple, half of my daughter's banana, and a string cheese. It occurs to me at this point that I'm having one of those "bottomless pit" days. My stomach continues to ask for more calories. "Remember all that walking you did today? And yesterday's run?" it says. Still, I've already had two snacks, and I'd rather get on with my afternoon and wait until dinner to eat again.

7:00 P.M. Good and hungry for dinner, I prepare a large meal of chicken burritos, brussels sprouts, brown rice, and a salad. After I finish my plate, I still have room for more. I eat what's left on my son's plate (waste not, want not) and finally feel satisfied.

DAY 1   DAY 2   **DAY 3**   DAY 4   DAY 5

7:15 A.M. The day started with fifty minutes on the elliptical trainer, my oatmeal breakfast, and decaf cappuccino with whole milk. I do seem to eat the same things over and over again, in spite of the dizzying variety of foods available. But I like my predictable routine. It's easy and comforting, and I don't have to think too much about portions. I know how these things make me feel, and I know I enjoy them.

12:30 P.M. I've eaten out quite a bit this week, so I'm really looking forward to preparing my favorite standard lunch at home. I eat a frozen chicken burrito from Trader Joe's that I microwave, then toast under the broiler because I love it crispy. I quickly assemble a small salad from some ready-to-eat lettuce, a few mushroom slices, and some crumbled feta cheese.

The dressing is simple: unrefined flaxseed oil and a nice balsamic vinegar shaken in a small container and tossed onto the salad. I'm still hungry when I finish both, because this standard lunch is typically not quite enough to fully satisfy me, so I generally add in a piece of fruit for dessert. Today it's a juicy navel orange because they're in season. My tummy feels just right. Satisfied and renewed, I'm ready to return to my work.

2:00 P.M. By midafternoon I'm hungry for a snack, so I eat a slice of whole wheat walnut bread with butter. It's barely noticed by my stomach, so I eat half a banana. Still hungry, I eat another small piece of walnut bread, this time with a modest wedge of goat's milk Brie. This is starting to look like a heavy snack, but my stomach wants it, and I know I won't be eating again until dinner, so I go for it.

8:00 P.M. It's date night, so we choose a nice restaurant within walking distance. Once we order our drinks, we ask the waiter to slow down the meal. Although I'm at 1 on the hunger scale, I prefer to stretch out and fully enjoy the eating-out experience. We eventually order the lamb shank entrée to share, which is an unusually rich choice for me, but we balance it with a vegetable side and rice. One entrée and two sides is the perfect amount for both of us. And then dessert appears. Warm apple tart with fresh whipped cream. Quite delicious. I finish at about 6 on my 10-point scale of fullness and leave the restaurant feeling relaxed and fantastic.

DAY 1   DAY 2   DAY 3   **DAY 4**   DAY 5

7:15 A.M. Oatmeal with fruit and my decaf, whole milk cappuccino. Nutrition, comfort, and routine to start my day.

8:30 A.M. The day begins with a step aerobics class at my gym. Yes, people still do step aerobics. I'm choosing to consider it a classic workout, rather than a failure to move on from my glory days of the eighties. Either way, it adds variety to my workout routine.

12:10 P.M. I check in with my stomach, and I'm hungry. I eat a chicken burrito, a small salad, and an orange.

3:30 P.M. I'm about a 1.5 on my hunger scale, so I eat my favorite whole wheat raisin bun with a smear of butter. I'm wanting more when I finish, but I'm not hungry enough. I know it will spoil my dinner if I eat more, so better to pass.

5:30 P.M. I eat one apple.

6:30 P.M. Tonight it's my daughter's favorite, Costa Rican Sausage Tacos (see "Full-Filling Recipes" at the end of the book). Already a bit hungry when I start, I peel a carrot and slice some fresh red pepper for me and my hungry kids to munch on while I get dinner on the table.

> I eat two corn tortillas topped with a quarter sausage each, cut into little bits, some of my homemade black beans that I pulled from the freezer, sautéed onion and pepper, and a bit of freshly grated sharp Cheddar. A dollop of salsa tops it off. I also steam a bag of pretrimmed green beans and add about 1 tablespoon of green goddess salad dressing. I'm not a fan of bottled salad dressing in general, but this one is natural and quite tasty as a veggie topping. I eat a bunch of green beans to get my fix of greens.
>
> I finish what's on my plate and find myself still wanting to pick, which means I'm still hungry, so I assemble and eat about a half taco more.
>
> My stomach doesn't clear later in the evening as I had expected it to. It's still digesting the tacos. Quick Re-Do. Notice the two-taco feeling in your stomach. That's the stop feeling. So I re-do the meal in my mind, stopping at two, knowing I have the option of a snack before bed if need be.

DAY 1   DAY 2   DAY 3   DAY 4   **DAY 5**

6:45 A.M. It's my scheduled high-intensity weight-lifting day, and I'm not up for it. I remember how much I have benefited from taking a rest day when my body wants it, so I do.

7:15 A.M. Instead of working out, I walk briskly over the big hill and down again to Peet's Coffee, my favorite. I order my decaf cappuccino "for here," which means it comes in a ceramic cup and saucer. Delightful on a sunny bench outside. I love this particular ritual.

9:00 A.M. My usual oatmeal and fruit.

12:15 P.M. There seems to be a rather large space in my stomach that would like to be filled. I eat my current favorite lunch, a chicken burrito and salad. A few of the season's first strawberries round out the meal. They aren't as good as I expected, but they will sit well with me and are the best option available, so I'm grateful for them anyway. I could eat more but decide to hold off so I can enjoy an afternoon snack.

2:45 P.M. I eat a whole wheat raisin bun with a thin layer of La Tur cheese, a delectable soft cheese that I brought home several days ago for a special treat. It is heaven.

7:00 P.M. I really don't want to cook, but one has to eat, and I'm quite hungry by now. I assemble the easiest meal I can manage: black beans, a bit of Spanish Manchego cheese, salad, and whole wheat couscous seasoned with sautéed onion, sun-dried tomatoes, and garlic, as well as a bit of olive oil. It does the job like an old Toyota. No style, no finesse, but it fills a need. I am delightfully satisfied. I go to bed with my stomach feeling just right, ready to collapse into a good night's sleep.

Progress Report

Over the next seven days, be sure to:

1. **Track your hunger before and after each meal.** In your Full-Filled Weight-Release Journal, begin keeping a hunger diary to help you get in touch with your body's signals of physical hunger and satiety. It will also help you identify the times and situations that are most likely to cause you to eat when you're not hungry or beyond the point of being full. Hunger is your body's natural signal that tells you when and how much to eat.

2. **Practice walking through the steps of the naturally slim and healthful eating strategy.** Decide what to eat based on true hunger and lasting gratification: the way the food will make you feel over time for the several hours that it is being actively digested in your body. With a little practice, you will notice yourself doing this almost automatically whenever you think about eating.

3. **Aim to reduce your intake of foods that contain ingredients that the body finds particularly confusing,** such as trans fats, high-fructose corn syrup, sugar, and artificial sweeteners, by 25 percent.

4. **Begin to replace refined, processed foods** with fresh produce (fruits and vegetables that are organically grown and free from hormones and pesticides), complex carbohydrates, lean protein, probiotics, and natural fats. Set an intention to reset your appetite for more healthful foods.

5. **Create a menu of standard foods and meals that you eat three times a day at regular times.** When your eating schedule is

predictable, your body anticipates when to digest food. This helps you manage your hunger and maintain or lose weight. Keep a record in your Full-Filled Weight-Release Journal of when and what you eat this week to help you establish a predictable routine.

6. **Begin to think of ways you can make your meals a ritual experience.** By making eating a ritual experience where the beginning and end of your meal is clearly defined and imbued with significance as a time for relaxation and renewal, you will find that you eat more mindfully and responsibly. This will positively affect your metabolism and weight.

7. **Begin to think of exercise as feel-good "me" time.** When you focus on the positive rather than the negative aspects of exercise and approach it as a feel-good activity with both immediate and long-term benefits, you'll want to do it more often. This week, determine the type of physical activity that makes you feel good. Maybe it's simply going for a walk around the block. Your body might love yoga, Pilates, or tai chi. Maybe it feels best on the basketball court or in the pool. Make a list of physical activities that make you feel good, and list them in your weight-release journal.

8. **Make a list of steps in small, doable increments that will get you moving.** Attach a date to each actionable step, including a date to start your new physical activity. If you don't currently exercise at all or if you exercise sporadically, getting into a routine will take some time and effort. Be patient with yourself, and as you tackle each of your steps, remain mindful of how fantastic you'll feel both immediately afterward and throughout the day.

Reliable, Long-Lasting Weight Release

Congratulations! You've made it to the final week of the Full-Filled program. Reflect with gratitude and appreciation on how far you've already come, and give yourself credit for the deep work you've accomplished. You've spent the past five weeks building a strong foundation for reliable weight release. Now it's time to top it off with a few additional concepts and tools that will allow you to maintain the positive behavior changes that you've made for a lifetime. What will really get you through the next six months . . . the next year . . . the next decade?

In Week 6 of the Full-Filled program, you will learn:

- How to practice the principle of continuous improvement
- The three Ps of positive change—persistence, patience, and practice
- How relaxed intent is so powerful for manifesting your dreams
- Why weight loss plateaus are gifts
- How to maintain a fulfilling life

Continuous Improvement

As you begin Week 6 of the Full-Filled program, **set your intention to take the tools and practices from this program deep into yourself, making space for continuous learning and**

improvement and great self-care. Let your intention arise and be present for you now.

In this final week, I will share my intention for you as well. My intent is to enable you to move clearly and fully into living your dream because I know that it's possible for you. I know you deserve it, and I know you can attain it.

In this final week of the Full-Filled program, I want to discuss a guiding principle in my work, a principle originally promoted by Dr. W. Edwards Deming in his Total Quality Management (TQM) system, which he taught back in the 1950s. It has everything to do with why Toyota is known for its quality cars.

You may wonder what building Toyota cars could possibly have to do with becoming naturally slim and healthy, and the answer is—an awful lot, actually. Building a quality car line and achieving reliable, lasting weight loss have the principle of *kaizen* in common. *Kaizen* refers to practices that focus on creating a state of continuous, incremental improvement. It's used most often in traditional fields such as manufacturing, engineering, business support, and management. With this process, the quality of Japanese cars dramatically exceeded the quality of cars coming out of Detroit in the 1950s. Because Toyota slowly and systematically improved its standardization and productivity over the years, its product eventually reached a point of reliability and superiority that made it almost impossible to beat.

As *kaizen* applies to weight release, the small shifts and changes that you've been noticing and appreciating internally and externally over the past five weeks have a similar effect. When you make continuous, consistent, and small incremental improvements day after day after day, you end up making big improvements that not only last but also keep getting better.

Notice that I said small incremental improvements. We're not talking about big breakthroughs here. Breakthroughs are wonderful and exciting, and you're likely to have had several over the past five weeks, but breakthroughs don't happen every day. As a culture, we've come to expect dramatic improvements at every turn. One of the most searched terms on the Internet is "fast weight loss." We want dramatic change, and we want it now! Our fervor and insistence for big change fast comes from a very strong away-from motivation. Remember away-from motivation? We hate our fat selves and want to move fast and far away from our flabby thighs. You know by now that this kind of motivation is short-lived at best and actually prevents you from making lasting progress.

Food for Thought

Give yourself credit for your progress along the way, however inconsequential it may seem. Over time, incremental improvements add up to breakthroughs and a lifetime of being naturally slim and healthy.

Kaizen takes the opposite approach. It lauds the small incremental steps and missteps because it recognizes that that's how significant progress is made. When you practice *kaizen,* instead of holding your breath for big breakthrough moments on the scale, a state of continuous improvement becomes your daily marker of success. You see, each of your day-to-day experiences is an opportunity for you to self-correct, learn, and improve. Remember, it's impossible to make a mistake that you can't learn from, so in the days, weeks, months, and years ahead, put yourself into a "learning state of mind" in which you recognize and appreciate that every experience in life affords you with an opportunity to learn and improve.

Kaizen, or continuous improvement, is the key to lasting and reliable progress, and I hope this principle provides you with a sense of comfort and relief. If you haven't come as far as you would like to by now, meaning you haven't slimmed down as much as you'd hoped, no worries. Progress happens in cycles, which is exactly how the Full-Filled program is set up. It's divided into six weeks of deep progress, where subtle changes begin happening as soon as day one and the long-term benefits extend far beyond the pages of this book.

Food for Thought

Kaizen means that you are mining your everyday experiences for areas where you can improve and areas where you can handle the situation just a little bit better next time. That means that when you overeat, you don't say to yourself, "Oh, I blew it, I might as well eat more and go all the way!" Instead, you say to yourself, "How can I use this experience as a springboard for improvement and positive change? What incremental improvement have I already made (remember the DIF), and what incremental improvement can I make from here forward?" When you make this shift, you will be amazed at how quickly your behaviors change.

So please don't beat yourself up if you aren't exactly where you want to be right now. Instead, accept and love yourself as you are today; take notice of and be grateful for the progress you've already made internally and externally. Then repeat the program, setting your intention to go deeper and release more. This may mean repeating certain steps of the program to get to a deeper layer of truth or release a limiting belief you might not have identified yet. Many people who follow the Full-Filled program cycle back through it several times while releasing more weight and then cycle through again to address and improve other areas of their lives, such as personal relationships or career and finance (remember: releasing limiting beliefs has rippling effects throughout all areas of your life). However you individualize your experience, the Full-Filled program allows for a continuous cycle of progress and reward.

Dig In: Review Your Progress

Refer back to your responses from the Dig In exercises in Week 1, notice how far you've come, and think about where you want to go from here. Review your away-from and towards motivations. This might be a good time to renew your short- and long-term motivation for the days, weeks, and months ahead.

Self-Correction and Kaizen

One of my favorite ways to integrate the concept of *kaizen* into the weight-release journey is by practicing the Re-Do. If you've been using this self-correction tool these past few weeks, you've already been practicing *kaizen* without even realizing it. If you haven't yet integrated this practice into your daily routine, I encourage you to find a regular time to do it, preferably in the evening just before you drift off to sleep, because that's such a malleable time for your subconscious mind.

Stretch out on your bed, and think back through your day. Ask yourself, "Is there any situation where I would like to do better next time?" By re-doing past situations and reinforcing new, healthful behaviors in your mind, you set yourself up for a pattern of continuous, compounding improvement. How great is that?

In addition to your nightly Re-Dos, I recommend getting into the habit of making a nightly Feel-Good List in your Full-Filled Weight-Release Journal. Now, before you whine, "More work? More lists?" let me assure you that this exercise is super quick (five minutes, tops; in fact, I bet you can do it in a minute or two) and the benefits dramatically outweigh any time investment you'll make. You will soon find that the few minutes you spend at bedtime not only become a comforting ritual but also boost your sense of daily satisfaction.

You may recall that I recommended the Feel-Good List as a

self-correction tool in Week 3, something you can do on your own to rebalance yourself energetically, emotionally, spiritually, and physically to get back on track to feeling good. To review, it's a quick, simple exercise in which you list one to two things from your day that make you feel good or that you're grateful for. That's it. Include anything that makes you feel really good when you think about it. It could be something as simple as enjoying your first morning cup of coffee or getting out the door on time for work, or it might be specifically related to your weight-release journey, such as self-correcting after a heavy lunch or putting your fork down when you're just satisfied. Generally, we get more of a feel-good hit from the small delights than the big ones, so when making your list, show gratitude for the simple moments in your daily life that you might often overlook as "trivial." Below are additional examples of "feel-good" moments that clients have shared with me:

- Connecting with a friend
- A smile from a stranger
- The sun shining
- Completing a project at work
- Being present with your child
- Feeling more relaxed around food that used to be a trigger
- Accepting a social invitation that, in the past, you would have passed on because you were embarrassed by your eating habits
- Doing something thoughtful or kind for someone "just because"

Your Feel-Good List can easily be incorporated into your Full-Filled Weight-Release Journal. Do not make the Feel-Good List an opportunity to judge yourself or your daily activities. Your intention is simply to take note of the moments in your day that made you feel good. The Feel-Good List works superbly to this end because by focusing on what's going right in your life, you inevitably put yourself into a positive state of mind. That's why making your list at night is so effective; your conscious mind is shutting down, and your subconscious mind is opening up. With regular practice, the Feel-Good List will retrain your subconscious mind to filter for the positive.

Whether you're aware of it or not, you're constantly filtering information into positive and negative categories. When I was a teenager, I learned that journaling was a good way to express emotions, so whenever I felt especially run down by my weight struggle and poor body image, I would pull out my journal and write about it. Though journaling helped me explore my emotions, I chronicled only the things that were going terribly wrong in my life. I was filtering exclusively for the negative! From time to time I'd go back and reread what I'd written in earlier journals and think, "I sound miserable!" In fact, my journals were filled with so much negativity that I eventually stopped the practice because it left me feeling more discouraged and disappointed in myself than ever. What I didn't realize was that filtering for the negative was only serving to keep me stuck in my weight struggle. I was magnifying my mistakes and minimizing my success. It was as if I had the telescope turned around the wrong way! No wonder I lost the motivation to keep up the practice.

It wasn't until I discovered the Feel-Good List, with its emphasis on filtering for the positive, that I started to chronicle my thoughts and emotions again and journaling became a positive experience for me. I'm not saying that writing about negative emotions is a practice you should avoid at all costs. Journaling in this way can help you slow down your thoughts and work through conflict and contentious relationships. As a general rule, however, I recommend that you end your entries on an upbeat note, and the Feel-Good List is a great reminder to do just that.

When you get into the habit of filtering for the positive right before falling asleep, you will inevitably start to notice and appreciate more positive experiences in your waking life. (Not only that, but you are also more likely to go to sleep on a positive note. Imagine how that will affect the quality of your sleep. And if you sleep well, imagine how refreshed and renewed you will feel when you wake up in the morning!) Once you start to become consciously aware of the positive moments marking your day, you will automatically adopt an attitude of gratitude that will attract more feel-good moments into your life.

Food for Thought

The positive feelings generated by the Feel-Good List will work their way through your subconscious mind, helping you discover more and more feel-good moments in your day. With regular practice, the Feel-Good List will create a new, automatic, positive filter that will support you in everything you do.

The Feel-Good List is so powerful that some of my clients actually believe it cured their depression.* Depression is all about the way we talk to ourselves and the thoughts in our heads. Depressed individuals filter for the negative in life, always seeing the cup as half empty. Having been depressed myself, I know how utterly impossible it can seem to feel good when you have your negative filters on.

The Feel-Good List is a simple, powerful way to retrain your thinking so that you filter for the positive. Add to that a self-renewing activity such as being in nature, listening to a favorite song, or enjoying a hot bath, and you have a great prescription for lifting your mood. (If slipping into depression is something you're prone to,

---

* This technique is not meant as a substitute for advice from a qualified medical professional. If you think you might be suffering from depression, do the Feel-Good List, and ideally some cardio exercise, and consult a qualified professional.

I also recommend good endorphin-boosting cardio exercise. Exercise has been shown to be at least as effective as prescription antidepressants in many cases; plus, you gotta love the side effects of exercise: better health and a firmer body!)

Someone Who Tried This Before You

Tami, a bright woman in her thirties, held a good job in corporate training and had already overcome a drug addiction when I met her. Still, she struggled with binge eating and depression. When she started my program, she believed that she would never be able to lose weight, attract a boyfriend, or successfully climb the corporate ladder. I recommended that she begin keeping a Feel-Good List.

I didn't see her for months afterward, but when I did, she told me that her whole life had changed. In the past, her to-do list at the end of the day had always left her feeling anxious and depressed, but once she started the Feel-Good List, she discovered that she ended the day on a positive note. She said, "You know, Renée, I'm a list maker, and before I started doing this positive exercise, I would go to bed thinking about my list and all of the many tasks that I hadn't completed. Now I go to bed and I think about all of the many tasks that I did accomplish in the day, and I feel great about that."

Instead of feeling bad about what she hadn't done, she retrained her brain to focus on the positive. Once she got herself into a more positive space on a daily basis, she was able to wean herself off antidepressant medication, lose 15 pounds, and revive her social life. A complete transformation!

The Three Ps of Positive Change

In addition to practicing self-correcting techniques such as the Re-Do and the Feel-Good List, you will continue to progress towards slim and healthy for a lifetime when you apply the three Ps of positive change:

Persistence

Patience

Practice

Persistence means that you will keep at it—practicing self-care, eating healthfully, and exercising regularly—day after day, month after month, year after year even through the occasional, or maybe the frequent, fumble. Because there's no such thing as failure, only feedback, when you screw up, you'll simply get back on course and move forward. What's made my *Inside Out Weight Loss* podcast work well for so many listeners is that they return week after week, tuning in for renewed support and motivation. In fact, some loyal listeners have been with me for more than two years. They listen to every new episode and cycle back through the older ones as a self-correction technique. Following the program has become part of their regular routine, and it's that persistence that has helped them make lasting, reliable progress.

Not long ago, a friend and I went to an exercise class in San Francisco, where I live, and the instructor was in phenomenal shape; she looked like a Jillian Michaels knockoff. She was slim, fit, and curved in all the right places. My friend asked me, "How does someone get a body like that?" and I replied, "A body like that does not come from a monthlong 'blitz' program. A body like that comes from years of persistence."

Though I can't compare my body to that instructor's, the reason I look as fit as I do for my height and build (and age!) is that I've been working at it since I was fifteen years old. Because of my ongoing persistence and dedication to exercise, my workouts today are less about overhauling and redefining my body and more about simply maintaining my current physique. When you develop an eating and exercise routine that makes you feel good while you're doing it (which is what you worked so intently on last week) and practice it consistently and persistently, reaching your ideal weight range and staying there indefinitely is not only possible but easy and enjoyable!

✔ Someone Who Tried This Before You

A successful business owner in Australia who was frequently asked to speak in front of large groups, Kimberly looked as if she had it all together. But in her personal life, she struggled. Twice divorced from abusive men, she swore she would never marry again. Added to that, she was 40 pounds overweight and suffered from a poor body image.

After several weeks of working with me, she discovered that her urge to overeat had significantly diminished. She was delighted. Several weeks later, however, her weight release stalled and she came to our session feeling stuck and discouraged. In our session, she expressed a concern that though her food consumption was down, her alcohol consumption had gone up, and she was suffering from feelings of shame and hopelessness. She said, "I worry that I'll be the one client of yours who fails the program. Maybe there really is something wrong with me, or maybe I just don't have what it takes to really change. Maybe I don't deserve it."

Despite her sense of defeat, Kimberly continued to show up for sessions in which she openly shared her fears with me. In other words, she persisted when the going got tough. We spent the time together identifying her limiting beliefs (can you spot them from the description above?) and transforming them into empowering beliefs that benefited not just her eating and drinking habits but also her personal relationships. In fact, partway through our coaching Kimberly met a kind and loving man, a totally different type from any of her previous relationships. About six months after our coaching sessions had concluded, she sent me beautiful wedding photos.

The second P of positive change is **patience**. It seems that most everyone with whom I work is impatient for results. When I ask, "How much weight do you want to release?" I often get answers like "If I could drop three pounds a week and release twenty-five pounds in the next two months, I'd be happy." More often than not, this is someone who has been overweight for ten or twenty years, and all of a sudden it's imperative that she take it off by tomorrow morning. The reality is that an urgent mind-set just doesn't work; in fact, it creates a level of psychological stress that is precisely the kind of emotion that makes us want to stuff our faces! Instead of falling into the hurry-up-now mind-set, be patient, focus on a journey of continuous improvement, and rely on your short-term motivators to pull you forward day after day after day. When you focus on the present and feeling good in your body each day with health-promoting practices, the future will take care of itself.

The third P of positive change is **practice**. Look at the masters in any discipline, the people who understand what it takes to be truly great at something. Think of a prima ballerina, an Olympic gymnast, a concert pianist, or anyone else who has gained mastery in a specific area. They didn't become masters without ongoing daily practice of their craft. In fact, it's said that it takes ten thousand hours of practice to truly master a discipline. That's certainly not overnight success, but we're often tricked into thinking it is because we aren't privy to the hours and hours of dedication and work that go into making a great, and oftentimes seemingly effortless, performance possible. Though it won't take you ten thousand hours to become naturally slim and healthy (insert sigh of relief; remember, you were born knowing when to eat and when to stop), the concept of learning through practice, with its mistakes and corrections, is the same for you.

Food for Thought

Persistence, patience, and practice. Practice what the Buddhists call nonattachment. Let go of the attachment to a number on the scale and practice doing something to promote your health and well-being each day, just like a true master. In this way, maintenance will take care of itself.

I have long required that clients who work with me privately make a six-week commitment to the Full-Filled program. I do so because I know that weight strugglers have a strong tendency to jump ship when the waters get choppy, typically when they are on the cusp of a major breakthrough. The temptation to give up when we're not getting the results we want fast enough can be very compelling, which is why persistence and continuous daily practice are so important to your progress.

I once had a client who said to me, "I feel like I'm always taking baby steps and I never really progress."

"Baby steps are ideal," I assured her, "as long as you continue to take them." Baby steps build on themselves, and before you know it, you've covered a lot of distance. Remember the compounding effect of *kaizen* and the success at Toyota? With practice and less time than you think, a walk will eventually turn into a jog, followed by a 10k run or even a marathon.

Running marathons used to be an activity reserved only for serious athletes, but these days, you'll find people of all ages, shapes, and sizes participating in marathons (I've seen nearly full-term pregnant women cross the finish line). To accommodate the increase in the popularity of the sport, many cities have marathon training groups in which amateurs (and by amateurs I mean first-time runners) learn how to run long distances. How can you learn to run 26.2 miles if you've never been able to huff it around the block? With slow and steady practice. I've known people who've completed marathons who before beginning to train for the race never owned a pair of running shoes! How does this happen? Did they just suddenly discover while training one morning that they were natural-born athletes? No. They were able to complete hours of intense pavement running in less-than-ideal weather conditions because they set small, achievable markers for themselves, such as running a block without stopping, that, once they reached them, they replaced with a new marker. After months of taking baby steps, they accomplished something they had never thought would be physically possible for them. Remember that forward momentum builds on itself. The only way to halt progress is to stop moving altogether.

Take a few moments now and make note in your Full-Filled Weight-Release Journal of how you plan to increase your persistence, patience, and practice over the next week and months, and imagine how stepping up the three Ps will help you in the face of setbacks.

Dig In: Persistence, Patience, and Practice

Ask yourself, "How can I increase my persistence, patience, and practice over the next several months? How can I increase my persistence, patience, and practice in the face of setbacks?"

Think back to what has thrown you off track in the past. Remember what I said at the beginning of this book? Every failed attempt you have made in the past has increased your knowledge of what doesn't work and therefore can contribute to your success today. It's time to harvest those lessons. Thinking back to the past, make a list in your Full-Filled Weight-Release Journal of the events that are most likely to throw you off track in the future—for example, vacations, deadlines at work, a sick child, a fight with your partner, a breakup, an illness, an injury. Now think back to your self-correcting techniques, and for each item on your list, ask yourself, "How will I continue to practice self-care and self-correction in these situations?"

If you find yourself resisting, that's good! You may be onto an undiscovered limiting belief. For example, if you think back to a crisis when you fell off the wagon and into the buffet line and think, "In that situation, all bets were off. I just had to survive," you may have an unresolved limiting belief that it's selfish to take care of yourself in that specific type of situation.

What if you believed instead that in times of extreme stress or crisis, renewing exercise could be what gets you through? I know I think that way, so when the going gets tough, I get moving because I know I especially need it then or I'll have nothing to give anyone else. I've exercised through my father's illness and death and through a crisis in my own marriage, and exercise was what got me through. Some days it was a simple walk through Golden Gate Park rather than a run, but I made sure I did something. Use the Emotional Freedom Technique to change any limiting belief you find, and then re-do the situation as you would like to have felt and behaved.

Complete this Dig In exercise by listing how you will self-correct for each item on your list, and then take a few moments to pre-do them in your mind. By patiently practicing persistence, you are deepening your transformation, increasing your mastery of naturally slim and healthful living, and creating your own insurance policy for future success.

Relaxed Intent

As you practice the three Ps of positive change, I want to throw another tool your way that's extremely important to manifesting your dream life. It will serve you well in the days ahead and as you cycle back through the Full-Filled program for additional benefits and insights. In the beginning pages of this book, I explained that setting intentions is like creating a blueprint or architectural plans for the reality you are creating. The concept of relaxed intent takes this a step further by adding an element of surrender and trust to your intention. Relaxed intent is based on the idea that when we relax about achieving a specific outcome, surrender the details, and trust that we will be okay whether or not we get it, change happens easily.

Have you ever noticed that sometimes when we really want something passionately, it's almost as if the very wanting of it prevents us from getting it? Let me give you an example of what I mean. Have you ever known a couple who really wants to get pregnant, and no matter how hard they try, even with the help of modern medicine, they cannot conceive? It's as if the very intensity of their desire prevents them from making it happen. Then, when they surrender their desire, perhaps by adopting, they become pregnant naturally. Or what about that good girlfriend of yours who really wants to fall in love? She puts herself out there, she dates, she puts endless energy into the whole process, yet every Friday night, she's still alone. Desperately wanting something and not getting it can be supremely frustrating. It runs counter to the Law of Attraction, which says you get what you think about most and direct your energy towards. I see this pattern happen again and again with weight loss. In fact, I've noticed that the people who have the greatest intensity, the greatest demand for change, are the ones who struggle the most. When a prospective client tells me she must lose weight fast, I know that she will be the one who gets the slowest results.

Confused?

I can almost hear your thoughts: "Renée, haven't you been telling me over the past five weeks to dream big and to stay motivated, determined, and focused towards becoming slim and healthy for a lifetime?" Yes, and now I must make an important clarification. Though it's important that you remain very clear about what you want for yourself, there's a big difference between demanding change and inviting change. A demand for change is when we must absolutely, positively have something, whereas an invitation for change is when we ask for what we desire, without the demand or desperation, and relax and open ourselves up to receiving it.

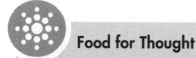

Food for Thought

Are you demanding change or inviting change? To answer this question, imagine accepting and feeling good in your body right now, as it is. If this throws you into a panic state—*No, no, no! I refuse to accept how I look and feel right now!*—you're demanding change. The giveaway is that you haven't accepted yourself unconditionally as you are right now. To get into a state of inviting change, go back to understanding the positive intent of why you eat and weigh what you do, and forgive yourself for wanting something positive for yourself. Appreciate the progress you've made, and surrender your desperate demand to be someone other than who you are right now. Bring your focus back to making the most of the present by choosing to feel good each day through nurturing, health-promoting behaviors. Change flows most easily when you are relaxed.

George Leonard and Michael Murphy wrote a book called *The Life We Are Given: A Long-Term Program for Realizing the Potential of Body, Mind, Heart, and Soul* about manifesting the intentions you set for your life. They introduce the concept of "focused surrender," in which you put yourself into a state of focusing on what you want while simultaneously surrendering your desire. It's not unlike the Buddhist principle of nonattachment, the process of letting go. "How does this work?" you ask. "How can I detach and let go of what I want and still get it?"

Although it's a silly example, I use the technique of detachment to manifest parking places. In San Francisco, finding parking is no easy feat. Spaces are beyond limited, and the minivan I drove for some years, often with a bunch of kids in it, carpooling them from one place to the next, didn't qualify as petite. I could have found parking difficult, but I've trained myself to get into a positive mental zone when looking for a place. I visualize finding a parking place within a block or two of the vicinity of where I'd like to have one, and then I tell myself, "That's what I want, but if I don't get it, I'll be all right. I'll find something a little farther away or go to a pay lot if need be. Either way, it's okay." I take a deep breath, relax, and mentally flip between getting the awesome parking place I want and not getting it. I go back and forth in my mind between having it and not having it and being fine either way. Nine times out of ten—I find the perfect spot. Even if I'm running late to meet someone or pick up a kid from school, I set my intention to practice relaxed intent, realizing that my heart will still beat and the earth will continue to turn if I don't find a space. It's really only when I don't cultivate a relaxed attitude and instead let myself reach a high-anxiety state of mind, circling the block and demanding to find parking, that a space never appears.

In *The Life We Are Given,* the authors relate a fascinating experiment concerning a gentleman named Duane Elgin of the Stanford Research Institute. He conducted a similar experiment, albeit much more scientific than my parking spot exercise, to test the power of intention. He utilized a magnetometer, a highly sensitive instrument designed to record changes or differences in magnetic fields on a moving sheet of paper, much as a seismograph records movements on the earth's surface. Elgin's idea was that with the power of his intention alone, he could influence the magnetometer. He hypothesized that if intention were real and he truly could focus his intention, he could certainly move the tiny, lightweight needle of the magnetometer.

He focused all the force of his will on the instrument for thirty minutes and watched the needle trace almost a straight line, indicating no change in the magnetic field. He did so again and again and again, and finally, exhausted and exasperated, he gave up. At the precise moment he "surrendered," the needle indicated a change in the magnetic field that was so significant that the needle went entirely off the chart. Elgin soon discovered that even physical distance didn't lessen the effectiveness of his intentionality when combined with his surrender. In one example, he was actually several miles away from the experiment site and was still able to influence the magnetometer at the precise moment of surrender. He concluded that it wasn't his intensity or focus but rather his relaxed intention and the act of letting go that produced the results he'd been after from the start.

So the question is: how does visualizing parking spaces and a spike on a magnetometer translate to weight release? When we think we must lose weight or our life will be unbearable, we're demanding to change. So if you think, "I must be slim to be happy," although you may think you're focused on what you want, you're actually focused on how awful your current body is and how desperate you are to change it. Desperation and anxiety are negatively charged emotions and only serve to attract more bad feelings your way. (And you know exactly what bad feelings trigger, don't you? Overeating.) The more you focus on "I must be slim to be happy," the less likely you are to become slim *or* happy. Your demand for change is a saboteur; it will undermine your noblest efforts to release weight and prevent you from moving forward towards a slim and healthy body.

 Food for Thought

A demand for change is when we must absolutely, positively have something, whereas an invitation is when we open our hearts—the doors of our soul—and our psyches to let in that which we desire, without demand or desperation but instead (notice the switch from the negative to the positive) with openness, relaxation, and surrender.

The key, then, to manifesting a slim and healthy body is first to focus on feeling good about yourself today (refer back to your Feel-Good List), then imagine what you want and invite it into your life in a relaxed, take-it-or-leave-it way. In other words, set a positive, relaxed intention around your weight release. Setting an intention brings you into a state of manifesting what you want in the present, especially if you're relaxed. (As a bonus, relaxation promotes speedier metabolism and all-around better health.) Be able to let go of the demand and need for what you want by focusing on the present and unconditionally accepting and loving yourself today, and mentally move back and forth between achieving your dream and not having it and being okay whatever the outcome.

Not sure how to relax? Take a deep, calming breath and sit back while I take you on a guided journey to help you create a state of relaxed intent.

 Mindful Meditation: Relaxed Intent

Take a deep breath, exhale, and let it go. You might even let it go with a nice audible sighing sound: "Ahhh." Now I want you to begin to think about what it is you really want. Think back to that dream body and life you imagined for yourself in Week 1 of the Full-Filled program. I wonder, has this image of your dream self evolved? You might be thinking about being in great health and having excellent mobility and loads of energy, and less about your actual pant size. Either way, hold the image of your dream self firmly in your mind, and then turn up the rest of your senses. What do you hear? What are your thoughts? How do you feel to be in that body, moving through the world? See yourself as a moving three-dimensional image, bright and vivid. See yourself clearly in your mind's eye, standing right in front of you. This is the object of your deepest desire, the "you" you've wanted to be.

Once you've made this image as real as possible in your mind, wrap your arms around it. Tense all of the muscles in your body, and hold on to the image of your dream self with everything you've got.

If it starts to slip away, grasp it even harder. Hold tight. Feel your want, your desire, and your demand for change. Hold on as long as you can, and then . . .

Let it go. Release it.

Feel the power of surrender, and watch the image of your dream self float away and dissolve into beautiful sparkles of light, which sprinkle down on you as thousands of tiny images of you, feeling happy and fulfilled in all different situations, in all different places, at all ages, in the future, and even in the here and now in your body today.

Notice that even after letting go, you're good. You already have so many blessings in your life. You're in a body that allows you to breathe, to listen, to feel, to move, to live, and, most important, to love. You're in the present moment, and you're okay just as you are. Linger in this positive state of relaxed intent for a few moments longer, and understand that by relaxing and letting go, you will manifest your dreams for the future in the present.

Throughout this final week of the Full-Filled program and in the days beyond, practice mentally moving between the desire to attain your dream and imagining what it would be like to let it go and completely accept yourself as you are now. What would it be like to honestly say, "If I don't have that, I'll be okay, maybe even good"? Let the attachment go, and feel good in your body and your circumstances right now. Esther and Jerry Hicks, who write extensively about the Law of Attraction, say, "The reason you want every single thing that you want, is because you think you will feel really good when you get there. But, if you don't feel really good on your way to there, you can't get there. You have to be satisfied with what-is while you're reaching for more." I love this quote because it speaks to the real "secret"—that in order to manifest all the things we want in our lives, we have to enjoy the process and the journey. And as we start to enjoy the ride, we realize that the true essence of what we want might just be the good feelings we experience along the way. Getting "there" then becomes a bonus to an already enjoyable journey. In other words, if you want to release weight so you can feel good about yourself, set an intention to feel good about yourself now, before you've released all your excess weight. That way you get to experience feeling good right away, and as a bonus, you'll feel even better when the excess pounds effortlessly disappear in the days, weeks, and months ahead.

Food for Thought

So many of us have been buying into what my friend Heather Dominick calls the "myth of arrival": "I'll be happy when I'm slim." "I'll be happy when I have a good relationship." "I'll be happy when I have more money." The Full-Filled program is all about enjoying the journey now. You can be naturally slim and healthy now, today, on the inside, and the outside will follow.

At any given moment, we never really know what serves our best interest; we just think we do. For example, when I was suffering from chronic fatigue syndrome, as far as I was concerned, life couldn't get any worse. Laid up in bed and unable to rally, I was forced to take time off from work, which made me feel like a financial burden to my husband and a slacker in the eyes of the professional world. I also had a newborn daughter whom I couldn't properly care for or attend to, so I felt like a failure in the parental department. I was miserable! Tangled up in self-loathing and guilt, I was not a woman who was appreciating the "journey."

Yet I was suffering from chronic fatigue for a very good reason: my body desperately needed a break. Because I wouldn't slow down, my body shut down on its own so that it would get the time it needed to realign and heal. In addition, my debilitation afforded me many hours to ponder my life. Eventually I came to understand that my chronic fatigue was directly tied to my weight struggle and the fears and limiting beliefs I'd held about myself for years. My self-worth was completely conditional on my body fat percentage and my professional achievements. That awareness gave my life new purpose: to release my own limiting beliefs and to develop a program that would help others release the root of their own weight struggle and begin living purposeful, fulfilling lives. Today I'm incredibly grateful for the journey. It was exactly what I needed at the time to guide me to where I am now.

If you choose, you can enjoy the journey even though you may not be exactly the weight you want to be. You can still enjoy how great it feels to take care of your body. You can still enjoy how great it feels to eat foods that make you feel wonderful over time. Today, enjoy the journey, and shift your intention from quick weight loss to healthful living. This is an intention that can be realized every single day, starting today.

Plateaus Are Gifts

I've described your weight-release journey as one of continuous learning and improvement. That said, understand that it won't always be a linear process. After releasing the root of your limiting beliefs in Week 4, you likely began to notice a shift in your weight (if you hadn't already). Perhaps you've dropped a noticeable amount by now. Or maybe you haven't experienced much of an external change yet. Either way, if you stay committed to the Full-Filled program—loving and accepting yourself as you are, practicing self-correction, reducing your DIF, releasing your triggers, eating to satisfaction, and making renewal and exercise part of your daily routine—you will eventually release all of your excess weight. And at some point, you may experience a weight plateau.

Oh no, the dreaded plateau!

I often think plateaus need a new PR rep because they get a terribly bad rap. When most people hit a plateau on their weight-release journey—meaning that their weight is stable for a day or a week or a month—they react negatively: "Oh my God, this is terrible. The world is ending. I'll never lose another pound." I've seen clients get so discouraged by this, but let's take a minute here and discuss what a plateau is. A plateau means you've lost weight and you're maintaining a weight lower than what your weight recently was. Did you get that? You're maintaining a weight lower than what your weight was. A plateau means that you have found thinner. Congratulations! This is what you've wanted all along—to maintain a lower weight, right? If you're maintaining at a slimmer level, your pants are probably looser. Maybe you're buckling your belt a little tighter. This is a good thing, yet hitting a weight plateau is often regarded as anything but. Why? Because most people interpret a plateau as a sign of failure, that their weight loss is slowing down, and that from this point on there will only be more effort and no reward. *I'm doing everything right, but the scale won't budge!* That's just not fair, now, is it? Hard work should produce results, and if your weight loss is leveling off, you might never reach that magic number on the scale. Our greatest fear is that our weight-release goals are ultimately unattainable.

Food for Thought

Just as a plane flying from San Francisco to New York never flies in a single straight line, your progress will not happen in a straight line, either. You will improve, then slip, then self-correct, and then be more successful the next time around. If you demand only improvement of yourself, you will quickly become discouraged, because growth doesn't happen in a straight line. Instead, be patient with yourself. Practice using the tools you've learned over the past six weeks. Allow your slip-ups to deepen your mastery, and in the long run you will be more successful.

Realize that weight release is a long-term, ongoing process and when you hit a plateau, it's important to use this break time to accept and enjoy how far you've come. You're smaller than you were before, and you alone created the change. Appreciate the accomplishment! Celebrate it by taking an indulgent walk in nature, sinking into a luxurious bath, or doing any activity that truly renews you. You've made progress. That's wonderful! Be sure to notice and enjoy how far you've come since starting your journey, rather than comparing yourself to how you want to be in the future. Remember: if you're enjoying the journey, the number on the scale becomes less important, anyway.

Understand that experiencing a plateau is a necessary part of the weight-release process. After releasing weight, your body needs to pause and readjust before it releases some more. Much as nature does throughout the winter months, your body's activity takes a rest. Not much is growing. The earth is brown and hard, and the trees are bare. Yet important things are happening beneath the surface. The plants and soil are resting and restoring. They are consolidating last year's growth and getting ready for the burst of life that is spring. The same can be said of you when your weight stabilizes in a plateau; your body is getting ready for the next period of great change and new growth.

Someone Who Tried This Before You

Liz came to me with only 10 pounds to lose, yet they were the same 10 pounds she'd been trying to lose off and on for twenty years. She had tried every weight loss plan and fad diet with no success and had finally come to me for a reliable solution. So we worked together, and, before she knew it, 5 pounds disappeared from her waistline. She maintained her new, slimmer weight for several weeks without losing a pound more. Though she was happy that the scale had finally moved, she wasn't through. She said to me, "Okay, I'm ready to take it to the next level. I want to get rid of the additional five pounds. What do I have to do?"

I said, "Well, let's look at your eating habits. What can we change now? Where would you like to be more at peace with food? Where would you like to feel even better?"

She'd already resolved one trigger situation—eating as a way to relieve boredom at work—so she dug deeper and discovered another trigger: she often overate at social events. By releasing and resolving that trigger, she was able to eventually drop the additional 5 pounds; yet it was the plateau that really got her there. The pause in her weight release gave her an opportunity to go deeper and identify where else she needed to shift her behaviors. The plateau enabled her to zoom in and tackle a very specific, unresolved trigger situation that had previously prevented her from reaching her ideal weight.

People who have significant amounts of weight to release often hit several plateaus along their weight-release journey. I once had a client who'd gotten down 135 pounds from her peak weight, and along the way she'd hit several plateaus. Each time she leveled out, we'd look at her current eating habits and identify where she was at peace with food and where she was still getting hung up.

Oftentimes, hitting a big milestone such as 100 pounds below your previous weight can trigger new fears and objections. Though releasing that much weight is a huge accomplishment, it can also feel scary. Clients often worry on an unconscious level about how their life might dramatically change, so they slow their weight release down. In this particular case, my client had some concerns about how her weight loss might affect her relationship with her husband. He wasn't used to having a wife who was slim and sexy, and she was used to being a woman who wasn't slim and sexy. She was a little nervous about how the dynamic between the two of them might change and how they'd adjust. Hitting a plateau after her milestone weight release gave her body a chance to catch up. It also gave her an opportunity to appreciate the present, update her identity, and readjust to the relationships around her.

Food for Thought

Slow, steady weight release is really a very positive thing because it allows your psyche, your spirit, your emotional life, and your identity to catch up with who you are, and who you're becoming.

Change happens in waves. Imagine your weight-release journey as a series of wavy lines. The peaks of the waves signify breakthrough moments when you release weight, and the dips, or the stretches between the peaks, represent the plateaus in your weight loss. Some weeks, you'll enjoy substantial weight release. Other weeks, you won't release any weight or might even gain a pound or two (gasp!). That's just how it goes, and this pattern is perfectly normal and healthy.

Plateaus are not signs of failure, but absolutely essential to reliable, long-lasting positive change. When you hit one, say to yourself, "I've hit a plateau. How can I fully enjoy the experience of being in a resting place, of consolidating the progress that I've already made? How can I fully appreciate my new, slimmer body as I prepare for the next phase? What more is there for me to learn here? Do I have an unresolved trigger that needs releasing?" Remember, plateaus are your body's way of stabilizing before it releases more weight. Be patient with your body, and while you are busy enjoying the present, the next wave will naturally occur.

Someone Who Tried This Before You

Simone, a warm, sweet woman in her late twenties, had a passion for performance. She was known as the life of the party and dreamed of moving to Los Angeles and making it in show business. She'd successfully dropped 30 pounds during our work together when her weight stabilized at just over 300 pounds. She was making great progress; she'd lost the urge to binge eat and drink in the over-the-top way she'd always done in the past. She had significantly reduced her DIF—the duration, intensity, and frequency of her overeating.

I explained to her that the plateau she'd hit was an opportunity for her to identify and release further objections she might have to being slim and healthy. I asked her to imagine herself 20 pounds lighter than she currently was, and she immediately crinkled up her nose at the thought.

"What is it?" I asked.

She replied that at 20 pounds lighter she would still be "huge and unhappy." Plus, she would have to face the fact that she'd let herself get so big in the first place, and she wouldn't have food to distract herself from her feelings of failure.

What Simone was really saying was that she still hadn't accepted herself as she was at that point, and without a foundation of self-acceptance, her weight release could go no further. As long as she hated herself for being "huge," she would never find herself truly worthy of self-care, and weight loss would always seem like punishment. Her weight plateau was her body's way of asking her for more love and acceptance.

We did some deep work to help Simone forgive and accept herself, yet her weight remained stable. She vacillated between feeling good about maintaining a lower weight and feeling discouraged that she wasn't "there yet." In one particularly emotional session, she said she wondered if it was even possible for her to be slimmer.

She said it felt as if she were in a hallway caught between two doorways. At one end of the hall was the doorway to her old self, and at the other end was the doorway to her slimmer self. When I asked her what prevented her from turning towards the door to her slimmer self, she said she felt she didn't deserve it. No wonder she couldn't release more weight! She had some serious limiting beliefs making the path forward inaccessible to her. I guided Simone through several rounds of the Emotional Freedom Technique in which she spoke her biggest fears out loud and released them.

Once she replaced her limiting beliefs with more empowering beliefs, the doorway to her slimmer self opened up. She checked in with me a couple of weeks later and shared that her temptation to snack had diminished further. She was releasing weight again, and, more important, she felt a new sense of compassion towards and acceptance of her current self that was truly liberating.

A final word on plateaus: when you set your intent to reach a certain weight, be sure to add, "this or something better" to your intention statement. For example, "I intend to release thirty pounds or something better." That way, you open yourself up to what's most healthful for you. When I was releasing weight, I had a very low number in mind that I wanted to reach, but my weight hit a plateau a few pounds before I reached it. I hovered at that weight for some time before I realized that it was actually the ideal weight for me. My target number had simply been too low. For me, the difference between being slim and healthy and being too thin and unhealthy was three pounds. Once I accepted that, I felt very happy with my weight and let go of my desire to drop lower.

The Full-Filling Life

As you finish the Full-Filled program or cycle back through it, set your intention to be on a lifelong journey full of learning opportunities and continuous improvement. Use the tools and practice the techniques that you have learned over the past six weeks to continue to evolve into a naturally slim and healthy person, and notice that in many ways you've already become that person. Appreciate that you've made significant progress, and feel gratitude for how far you've come. Notice all the blessings in your life, and take time to enjoy your body and your life today. Because a continuous cycle of improvement is what the Full-Filled program is all about, if something happens in the days, weeks, or months ahead that sets you two steps back or throws you off course, simply self-correct, give credit to the learning process, feel empowered, and trust in the journey; then, if you choose, dive back into the program and go deeper for additional benefits and insights. Continue to cycle through the entire six-week program, or simply repeat certain weeks until the concepts and practices are part of your daily routine and ritual.

Someone Who Tried This Before You

Lee, a client of mine, was a bulimic when we started working together. After following my program for several months, she came to see me one afternoon and reported that for several weeks straight she hadn't binged. I said, "Congratulations. You've made huge progress. What do you think about spacing our sessions out to every two or three weeks now since you're doing so well on your own?"

The idea that she wouldn't spend as much time thinking or working on her weight struggle made her nervous. She said, "My weight struggle has been so intense and constant for so long, it feels disorienting to think about it taking a backseat role in my life." She was actually starting to feel a void where her weight struggle had been.

I told her, "This is a good problem to have; you're not good at bingeing anymore, you've reduced your duration-intensity-frequency, and you're waking up to the rest of your life. That's great news! Now let's turn our focus to the part of coaching I love the most: discovering and developing your unique gifts."

Lee had been consumed by her weight struggle for so long that she'd forgotten what else interested her, so I asked her to think about what brought her enjoyment. Though it took her a few moments to respond, eventually she came up with two things that would make her quite happy. Number one on her list was to develop deeper connections with a few of her valued friends. She started scheduling hikes with friends and also showing up to social engagements that she would previously have blown off. Her friends were surprised and delighted to see more of her. The second item on her list was to be more creative. She really enjoyed scrapbooking, so she started setting aside time to devote to her favorite hobby. She could hardly believe how rewarding it felt to have the time and energy to nurture her relationships and engage in activities she enjoyed doing!

Now it's your turn. What do you dream of replacing your weight struggle with? Do you dare to dream? I encouraged you to begin exploring what you'd like to reintroduce into your life at the end of Week 4. What did you come up with? What activities appeal to you? What do you enjoy doing most? Do you have hobbies you want to pursue?

Ending the weight struggle and coming to peace with your body and your life will free up so much of your time and allow you to rediscover who you really are. I've had clients who have taken up activities as diverse as hot-air ballooning, knitting, kayaking, competitive racewalking, volunteering at a local nonprofit, and simply spending more time with friends and family. What is it that you would like to experience for the first time or do more of? I once asked my *Inside Out Weight Loss* podcast listeners what they planned to do once their weight struggle no longer had a hold on them. Here are some of my favorite responses:

"I'll replace my weight struggle with discovering what else life has to offer. I'll roller-skate and dance!"

"I want to replace my struggle with contentment for who I am and what I look like today. I've never been comfortable with me. I've never accepted myself for who I am. If I can make that shift, I can do anything."

"I want to replace my obsession with food and weight with more meditation time and gratitude and generosity towards others."

"I'd like to replace my weight-release struggle with renewed energy and happiness. With three kids, I want to be able to play and have fun with them without even thinking of it being work or physically exhausting."

"The sweet spot in my day will no longer be food but the connections I make with other people. That's what I want to focus on and enjoy most."

"I dream of, and fully expect, to be more and more kind to myself when I sit down to eat. And I expect this kindness at meals to influence the rest of my life. Not all by tomorrow . . . but gradually and permanently."

When you no longer use food as your go-to pastime, your crying rag, your best friend, or your lover, you will find that other things move into your life to occupy that space. Activities and experiences that hold more enjoyment than food ever has will begin to fill out your life. Suddenly the bright spot in your day will not be the cupcake from the bakery down the street but the smile on your child's face and the bright sunlight you feel on your own cheeks.

As you imagine all that life has to offer, sink into the following mindful meditation "Replace Food as Your Best Friend."

Mindful Meditation: Replace Food as Your Best Friend

Take several deep breaths and sink into a state of relaxation. As you do, I want you to begin to think about food: your cravings for it, your enjoyment of it, your attachment to it. Create an image in front of you. It may be of a particular type of food, it may be of multiple foods. Whatever it is, notice how this food makes you feel. What does it represent to you? Comfort? Relaxation? Distraction? Entertainment? Do you think of food as your constant and reliable best friend, as a bright spot in the middle of your day? Feel the pull and attraction of food, and as you do, notice the brightness it has.

Now imagine the food in your mind's eye becoming dimmer and falling away from the brightness. In its place, imagine other things moving into the spotlight. Bright and sparkling, they move in and occupy that place in exactly the same way that food used to. Those other things may be clearly defined, or they may not. Take your time here, and imagine that the light that shone so brightly on food for so long now illuminates other areas in your life, such as making mean-ingful connections with people, expressing your creativity, being generous to those you love, finding reasons to laugh, or whatever else it is that feeds your spirit.

Notice the light naturally emanating from these many new areas in your life in a way that it never did with food. Imagine that light expanding and radiating outward and then back towards you, bathing you in a warm, beautiful glow from the outside in and the inside out. Imagine moving through the days, weeks, months, and years ahead feeling nurtured and renewed by the relationships and activities you participate in now that you're free from the weight struggle.

As you come to the end of Week 6 of the Full-Filled program, I wish to express my heartfelt gratitude to you for allowing me to lead you on this journey. It is a privilege and a joy to me that my life's work is helping you. Thank you for giving me the opportunity. If there is only one message that you take away from this experience, I want it to be this: no matter how long you have struggled, no matter how much excess weight you have carried, your struggle does not define you. You are more than your struggle, you are more than your weight, and you can truly be who you want to become.

Positive change is possible, and it's possible for you. I know this because I have risen from the depths of my own despair and have seen others rise from circumstances far more challenging than mine. They used the transformative tools you now hold in your hands to live lives they had never thought possible. Now it's your turn to create a truly fulfilling life for yourself. This is my dream for you.

Progress Report

Over the next seven days, be sure to:

1. **Appreciate and celebrate the progress you've made over the past six weeks.** Refer back to your responses to the Dig In exercises from Week 1, notice how far you've come, and think about where you want to go from here. Review your away-from and towards motivations, and renew your short- and long-term motivations for the days, weeks, and months ahead.

2. **Start a Feel-Good List in your Full-Filled Weight-Release Journal, and begin to train your mind to filter for the positive.** Simply list one or two things from your day that make you feel good or that you're grateful for. They could be something as simple as enjoying your first morning cup of coffee, or they might be specifically related to your weight-release journey, such as self-correcting after a heavy lunch or putting your fork down when you're just satisfied. You will soon find that the several minutes you spend chronicling your feel-good moments will not only become a comforting ritual but also boost your sense of daily satisfaction.

3. **Integrate the three Ps of positive change into your long-term maintenance plan.** Note in your Full-Filled Weight-Release Journal how the three Ps—persistence, patience, and practice—will help you practice self-care, eat healthfully, and exercise regularly over the weeks and months ahead. Note also how you will self-correct through setbacks with persistence, patience, and practice.

4. **Set a positive, relaxed intention around your weight release.** Flip between the desire to attain your dream and imagining what it would be like to let it go and completely accept and feel good about yourself as you are now. Set aside at least five minutes this week for the mindful meditation "Relaxed Intent." The key to manifesting a slim and healthy body is to let go of your demand and need for what you want and feel good about yourself today, then imagine what you want and invite it into your life in a relaxed, take-it-or-leave-it way.

5. **Set your intention to be on a lifelong journey full of learning and continuous improvement.** Use the tools and practice the techniques that you've learned over the past six weeks to continue to evolve into a naturally slim and healthy person. Appreciate that you've made significant progress, feel gratitude for the blessings in your life, and take time to enjoy your body and your life today. Continue to cycle through the entire six-week program, or simply repeat certain weeks until the concepts and practices are part of your daily routine.

Full-Filling Recipes

To give you an idea of what dishes make my life easier and more pleasurable, I've included several of my favorite recipes and snacks for you to try.

Breakfast

Quick and Natural Oatmeal

I have long loved oatmeal. It's warm, nutritious, and filling. When I'm organized, I will set up the rice cooker the night before with steel-cut oats so they are ready for breakfast. More often, however, I make rolled oats in the microwave in the morning. I advise against the individual serving packets of oats, as they are typically made with instant oats, the most processed kind, and have all sorts of other undesirable ingredients in them, such as sugars and artificial flavorings.

Plain old rolled oats are cheaper and actually very easy to prepare. The key for microwave preparation is to use a very large bowl, as they expand tremendously during cooking and will spill over in a smaller bowl.

This is my typical serving, which is light for me, but leaves me nice and hungry for lunch or a midmorning piece of fruit if need be.

Serves 1

¾ cup rolled oats

1½ cups water

1 tablespoon live yogurt, unsweetened (I prefer yogurt made
   from whole milk)

2 walnut halves

Fruit of your choice

Combine the oats and water in a large, microwave-safe bowl. Microwave on high for 4 minutes, or until all the water is absorbed. Serve
with yogurt, walnuts, and a fruit of your choice. My favorites include
either ½ orange or 8 to 10 grapes.

Banana Smoothie

This is a superfast, yummy breakfast or snack for warm weather. I
adapted it from a recipe from the Jena Wellness Center in New York
City.

Serves 2

2 ripe bananas (or frozen bananas for more coolness and texture)

2 cups milk of choice (cow's, almond, soy, rice, etc.)

1 tablespoon almond butter

1 cup ice cubes

½ teaspoon cardamom

½ teaspoon coriander

Cinnamon for sprinkling

OPTIONAL

1 scoop unsweetened protein powder

Add all the ingredients to a blender and blend until smooth. Deco-
rate with an extra sprinkling of cinnamon at the end.

Favorite Protein-Fruit Smoothie

(Inspired by my pal Gina Orlando, who always has
a tasty recipe up her sleeve)

Protein digests more slowly than carbohydrates, so a high-protein breakfast is a good choice for extending enjoyment and satisfaction throughout the morning. I think you will find that the natural sweetness of the fruit is more than enough once your taste buds are reawakened to the delicious subtleties of natural food.

Serves 1

1 cup water
½ cup frozen mango cubes
½ cup frozen berries (strawberries, mixed berries, or blueberries)
1 scoop (5 tablespoons) protein powder (egg white, whey, or rice protein)
1 tablespoon flaxseed oil (omega-3 fat), or 1 to 2 teaspoons freshly ground flaxseed (The ground seeds add fiber as well as omega-3 fats. Some people with nut allergies can be sensitive to flax. Most people do fine with it.)

OPTIONAL
1 teaspoon fiber (ground flaxseed, mixed fibers, or psyllium or ¼ teaspoon apple pectin) if you don't add the ground flaxseed. (Fiber will make it grittier, but can help clear your intestines and eliminate toxins. If you bloat after taking fiber, try a different kind or less of it.)
1 to 3 teaspoons superfood/green powder (freeze-dried veggies, algae, and fruits; some also contain probiotics)

Blend and enjoy!

Simple Toasty Breakfast

I really enjoy the simple pleasure of good whole grain bread with a bit of real butter. As fat is digested more slowly than protein, this combo usually takes me through the morning. My favorite kind of bread is sprouted grain, as it retains most of its nutrients and has a subtle, nutty flavor.

Serves 1

2 slices sprouted grain bread, sprouted bagel, or whole wheat
   English muffin
1½ to 2 teaspoons butter
1 piece whole fruit or sliced melon (fresh fruit is a great
   substitute for sugary jam)

Toast the bread as desired, and spread with butter. Enjoy with fruit on the side or on top.

Variation
For the butter, substitute 1 tablespoon peanut butter, a few slices of fresh avocado, cottage cheese, or even yogurt.

Egg Toasty Breakfast

No list of breakfast options would be complete without eggs!

Serves 1

1 slice sprouted or whole grain bread
1 teaspoon butter
2 eggs, any style

OPTIONAL
1 to 2 tablespoons salsa
Fresh fruit

Toast the bread as desired, and spread with butter. Enjoy with eggs. Increase the heat and fiber with a tablespoon or two of salsa if desired. Enjoy with a piece of fresh fruit if you like.

Lunch

Salmon Salad

This quick and easy salad is ideal for packing to go. I put the dressing in a small refrigerator container and put it in with the salad, so if it leaks, it leaks on the salad. Canned bone-in, skin-on salmon is rich in omega-3 essential fatty acids, as well as loaded with calcium from the soft, edible bones, making this lunch a nutrition bonanza and perfect for helping you feel great all afternoon.

Serves 1

About 3 cups dark lettuce or fresh spinach
A few mushrooms, sliced
A few cherry tomatoes
1 tablespoon crumbled feta, blue, or goat cheese
1 tablespoon olive oil plus 1 teaspoon balsamic vinegar,
    combined
½ (7.5-ounce) can bone-in, skin-on salmon

Combine the veggies and cheese. Toss with oil and vinegar and top with the salmon. Add a piece of whole grain bread or ½ cup brown rice if you'd like to round out the meal with some carbs.

Vegetarian Option
For a vegetarian option, substitute 2 hard-boiled eggs or some seasoned baked tofu for the salmon.

Corn Quesadilla

This easy lunch can be made at home in a frying pan or at work in a microwave. Serve with a small salad, such as the Salmon Salad, omitting the salmon.

Serves 1

Spray oil
2 corn tortillas, or 1 whole wheat tortilla
½ cup frozen corn
About ½ cup grated cheese

Stove-top instructions: Heat a frying pan and spray with oil. Add a tortilla and heat until just warm. Flip and spread with the corn, then the cheese. Top with the second tortilla or fold the wheat tortilla in half, covering the cheese and corn. When the cheese has melted slightly, flip and heat through until the cheese has melted and the tortilla has golden-brown patches.

Microwave instructions: Place a tortilla on a microwave-safe plate. Top with the corn and cheese. Cover with the second tortilla or fold the wheat tortilla in half. Microwave on high until the cheese has melted, 1 to 2 minutes depending on the microwave.

"Prosocial" Black Beans and Rice with Salad
(Again, inspired by my pal Gina Orlando)

In my opinion, fresh beans are the ultimate health food. Naturally low in fat but high in fiber and nutrients, they are a staple in my diet. Beans and rice make a great workday lunch when paired with a small salad or other vegetable.

Making beans from scratch can seem daunting, but it's actually quite easy because the prep time is minimal. I often set a batch of beans to soak on Friday or Saturday night, then simmer them the following day while I go about household chores. If I make a double batch, I freeze half to use in Costa Rican Sausage Tacos (see page 293) or to serve for dinner with brown rice and roasted vegetables at a later date.

The other great revelation I've had, courtesy of the Weston A. Price Foundation (www.westonaprice.org) and my friend Gina, is that the addition of unfiltered apple cider vinegar partway through the simmering process removes most of the unsocial gas-producing effect of beans, making this a "prosocial" recipe!

Serves 6 or more, depending on portion size

1 pound dried black beans
8 cups water
1 whole bay leaf
4 cloves garlic, minced
⅓ cup extra-virgin olive oil
1 cup red wine
1 red or green bell pepper, diced
1 tablespoon ground cumin
1 tablespoon dried oregano, or 2 tablespoons chopped fresh
   oregano
¼ teaspoon cayenne pepper
1 to 2 tablespoons unfiltered apple cider vinegar
2 teaspoons salt

Rinse the beans and remove any damaged beans or stones. Cover with water to 2 inches above the beans. Allow to soak at least 8 hours or overnight.

Discard the bean-soaking water, and add 8 cups water. Bring slowly to a simmer (about 45 minutes), stirring occasionally, and skim off any residue at the top of the water. Simmer for an additional hour. Skim again if necessary.

Add the remaining ingredients except for the salt and bring back to a simmer. Cook for another 45 minutes or so, until the beans are soft but still hold their shape. Towards the end of cooking, add the salt (adding it earlier toughens the beans).

Brown Rice

If you don't own a rice cooker, consider investing in one that can make brown rice. With it the rice comes out perfect every time, and it's supereasy. The fancier ones will let you set up the ingredients well in advance and have them ready when you want. This feature also makes preparing steel-cut oats (the most whole grain kind) a snap because you can set up the rice cooker the night before and have steaming oats ready for breakfast.

I consider brown rice to be a different food from white rice. Though long-grain white rice is preferred by the Western palate, long-grain brown rice can feel sharp. I prefer short or medium grain for the chewy and smooth texture.

Serves 2 to 3

1 cup short-grain or medium-grain brown rice
2½ cups water
1 tablespoon unfiltered apple cider vinegar

Combine all the ingredients and let them soak for 6 hours. This will make the rice more digestible, just like the beans. You can skip the vinegar and still have great rice, but adding it makes it even better. The rice will not have a vinegar flavor, by the way, as it cooks off.

Bring to a simmer, and simmer covered to desired softness, 45 to 50 minutes.

Serve the black beans and brown rice with a salad or another vegetable side. Top with creamy yogurt or a bit of grated sharp cheese, or add a splash of balsamic vinegar for a bit of zip if desired.

Dinner

10-Minute (or Less) Weeknight Salad

This salad is fast, easy, and packed with nutrition. I probably make it four times every week. When I serve it at dinner parties, every last leaf is eaten. The raw garlic adds loads of flavor and is a great antiviral. I've been known to put in 3 or more cloves when someone needs an immunity boost. Just make sure everyone eats some!

Serves 2 to 4

SALAD
½ (6-ounce) bag ready-to-eat organic spinach, romaine, or other salad greens
1 carrot
A handful of fresh mushrooms, sliced
⅓ cup crumbled feta cheese

OPTIONAL
Sliced fresh red pepper
Cherry tomatoes, tossed in whole or cut in half
Slices of cucumber
2 tablespoons defrosted frozen peas
1 tablespoon chopped walnuts or pecans

DRESSING
2 tablespoons extra-virgin olive oil
1 tablespoon balsamic vinegar
1 clove fresh garlic, unpeeled

Put the lettuce in a large bowl. Peel the carrot. Continue to use the vegetable peeler to peel off slices of carrot directly into the bowl. This creates light bits of carrot that add color and flavor but do not sink to the bottom of the salad. Add the other veggies, the cheese, and the nuts.

Combine the oil and vinegar in a small jar with a lid, such as a plastic storage container or an old jar. Place the clove in a garlic press, and press the garlic directly into the oil and vinegar. Put lid on the jar and shake to combine. Pour over the salad and toss.

Yum!

One-Pot Chicken Stew

This is an easy, tasty chicken stew I make for my family. I make a double batch to last for three or four meals and pair it with a salad and whole grain bread. We are not big meat eaters in my family and tend to use meat more as an accent flavoring, so this is one of the meatier recipes I make. Even so, we generally eat one drumstick per person, per meal. I prefer organic chicken because the chickens are treated more humanely, and I like to avoid meat that has been treated with antibiotics and growth hormones. I also prefer dark meat for its fuller flavor. You could just as easily make this recipe with chicken breast if you prefer. But leave the skin and bones on, because that's where all the flavor comes from, and the amount of added fat is small. Don't eat the skin, just cook with it.

This recipe calls for broccoli florets. You can substitute another green—chopped chard or kale or even halved brussels sprouts, for example. The green vegetable, which is alkaline, nicely balances the acidity of the tomatoes.

Serves 5

1 tablespoon olive oil

1 (5-piece) package chicken drumsticks or thighs, bone in and skin on, or chicken breasts if you prefer

1 large onion, chopped into bite-size pieces

3 medium potatoes, chopped into bite-size pieces

3 medium carrots, peeled and chopped into bite-size pieces

1 (14-ounce) can chopped tomatoes

1 (25-ounce) jar pasta sauce

½ cup water

A handful of chopped fresh basil, if available, or 1 tablespoon dried basil

4 cloves garlic, minced

1 package broccoli florets, or the florets from one bunch of broccoli

Freshly ground black pepper to taste

Heat a large Dutch oven on medium-high. When the pan is hot, add the olive oil and swirl to coat the bottom of the pan. Once the oil is hot, add the chicken pieces and brown, stirring occasionally, about 5 minutes.

Add the onions, potatoes, carrots, and chopped tomatoes. Add the pasta sauce, then add the water to the empty pasta sauce jar, swirl it around to get the last bits from the jar, and pour into the pot. Stir well, reduce heat to low, and let heat through, about 10 to 15 minutes.

Add the basil, garlic, and broccoli, and stir well. Let simmer until chicken is cooked through, about another 20 minutes. Add pepper to taste.

This stew's flavor will improve if left to sit for an hour or two before serving and will taste even better the next day.

Quiche—Kid-Friendly Version

(Adapted from *The Moosewood Cookbook*, by Mollie Katzen)

I normally make about four of these quiches at a time. They freeze pretty well and keep for about four days in the fridge.

Serves 4

1 tablespoon butter
1½ cups chopped onion
½ teaspoon sea salt
Black pepper to taste
A pinch of thyme
½ teaspoon dry mustard
4 medium eggs
1½ cups whole or 2% milk
2 tablespoons organic unbleached flour
1 (10-inch) frozen whole wheat pie crust made without
   hydrogenated oils (available at health food stores)
1½ cups loosely packed grated aged hard cheese, such as a good
   Gouda or Cheddar (you can substitute about ¾ cup cubed
   Brie or mix bits of leftover cheeses)
Paprika for sprinkling

Preheat oven to 375 degrees F.

Melt the butter in a frying pan. Add the onions and sauté over medium heat for a few minutes. When they begin to soften, add the salt, pepper, thyme, and mustard. Sauté about 5 minutes more and remove from heat.

In a blender, combine the eggs, milk, and flour and beat well. Spread the onions over the base of the pie crust. Top with the cheese. Pour in the egg mixture and sprinkle with paprika.

Bake for 35 to 45 minutes, or until solid in the center.

Variation 1
Instead of the pie crust, use 4 corn tortillas arranged like a crust on the bottom of a pie pan.

Variation 2 (adult friendly)
Sauté 6 ounces fresh spinach with 1 teaspoon butter or oil and 2 cloves chopped organic garlic until just wilted. Add to the pie crust with onions and top with the cheese.

California Shepherd's Pie

Shepherd's pie is a traditional English casserole-style dish, typically featuring a base of ground meat with the odd vegetable and plenty of Worcestershire sauce, topped by rich mashed potatoes. As it's a favorite of my British husband, I adapted the concept to suit a more California-style (veggie lovers) taste. Here the meat is used more as a flavoring than as the main feature of the meal.

Serves 10

POTATO TOPPING
4 pounds Yukon Gold potatoes, chopped into large chunks for boiling (the smaller the chunks, the quicker they cook)
1 tablespoon plus 1 teaspoon sea salt
1 cup whole milk
1 tablespoon butter
1 teaspoon freshly ground black pepper

"PIE" BASE
Spray oil
2 tablespoons oil such as grape-seed, peanut, canola, or other mild oil for sautéing
2 onions, chopped
2 carrots, peeled and chopped into bite-size chunks

2 tablespoons dried cumin

3 organic zucchini, chopped into bite-size chunks

6 large cloves organic garlic, chopped

1 pound ground turkey

2 (15-ounce) cans cannellini beans, drained

1 (15-ounce) can chopped tomatoes or more to taste

A handful of fresh basil, chopped

Paprika for sprinkling

OPTIONAL

1½ cups grated hard cheese, such as Cheddar or Romano

Preheat oven to 350 degrees F.

Bring a large pot of water to a boil. Add the potatoes and 1 table-spoon salt and bring back to a low boil. Cook for approximately 20 minutes, or until the potatoes are tender, and drain off most, but not all, of the water.

While the potatoes are cooking, coat a roasting pan with spray oil. Heat about 1 tablespoon of the oil over medium heat in a large frying pan. When the oil is warm, sauté the onions, carrots, and cumin until the vegetables are just tender, then pour into the roasting pan. Add a bit more oil to the frying pan and sauté the zucchini until crisp-tender, then add to the roasting pan. Add a bit more oil to the frying pan. When the oil is warm, add the garlic and sauté for about a minute. Add the turkey meat and sauté until not quite cooked through, then add it to the roasting pan. Add the beans, tomatoes, and basil to the roasting pan and mix all the ingredients well.

Heat the potatoes over medium heat and add the milk, butter, remaining salt, and pepper. Mash the potatoes, adding more milk if needed to achieve a smooth consistency.

Spread the potatoes over the vegetable-turkey mixture. If using cheese, spead evenly on top. Sprinkle with paprika, then bake for about 40 minutes, or until the edges bubble.

Lentil Stew

Lentil stew is a family favorite. It's quick to prepare, as the lentils take only about 20 minutes to cook. I can make a huge pot in about 45 minutes, and it will last the family for several days. Plus it's a nutritional powerhouse! Note that lentils are less gas-producing than other legumes, an important selling point!

Serves 6

½ to 1 gallon water, depending on how thick you want the stew
3 cups brown lentils
2 baking potatoes, or 4 smaller potatoes cut into bite-size chunks
3 carrots, peeled and cut into bite-size chunks
2 large yellow onions, cut into bite-size chunks
2 bay leaves
2 bunches chard, chopped
1 (28-ounce) can chopped tomatoes
6 cloves garlic, chopped
1 tablespoon Asian fish sauce, or 2 teaspoons salt
1 tablespoon cumin
1 teaspoon sea salt or more to taste
Grated fresh ginger to taste (start with 1 tablespoon)
Freshly ground black pepper to taste

OPTIONAL
2 precooked chicken or turkey sausages, chopped
Whole milk plain yogurt for dolloping on top of each bowl
Fresh parsley or other herb for garnish
Grated aged hard cheese

Put the water, lentils, potatoes, carrots, onions, and bay leaves into a large pot. Add water if necessary to cover all the ingredients by about 2 inches. Bring to a boil and immediately reduce to a simmer. Cook for about 10 minutes and add the chard. When the chard has wilted, add the tomatoes, garlic, fish sauce, cumin, sea salt, ginger, pepper, and optional sausages. Continue cooking until all the ingredients are tender, about another 15 minutes. Adjust seasoning to taste.

Serve with a dollop of whole milk plain yogurt or the shreds of a good aged, hard cheese. Add a sprig of parsley or another fresh herb if you really want to get artistic.

Healthful Tortilla Pizza

This is healthful fast food for one or a family. If you have kids, they can learn to make their own, adding any additional desired toppings, such as leftover vegetables or even a few slices of pepperoni.

Serves 1

1 whole wheat tortilla, about the size of your largest frying pan
¼ cup pasta sauce
1 ounce mozzarella cheese, grated

Heat the pasta sauce in the microwave for 45 seconds on high.

Heat a large frying pan over medium heat. Place the tortilla in the pan. When it is warm and slightly crisp, flip it to the other side. Spread the pasta sauce over the tortilla and sprinkle with the grated cheese. Heat until the cheese has melted.

If you are making more than one pizza, crisp the tortillas in a 425 degree oven instead of using a frying pan, add the topping, and return to the oven to heat through and melt the cheese.

Pork Tenderloin Agrodolce

(Adapted from *Cooking Light*, November 2010)

For the longest time I didn't eat pork, and I'm not sure why. I think it was the pork industry's campaign telling us that it's "the other white meat" that made me reconsider when I was looking for some variety in my diet. I'm glad I did, as this recipe has become a family favorite.

Serves 8

¾ cup balsamic vinegar
½ cup dried cranberries or cherries
¼ cup chicken broth or water
1 tablespoon sugar or 1½ teaspoons honey
6 cloves garlic, chopped
3 thyme sprigs, chopped
1 pound cipollini (short, flat) onions, slightly chopped (substitute yellow onions if cipollini aren't readily available)
1 teaspoon kosher salt
2 tablespoons extra-virgin olive oil
2 (1 pound each) pork tenderloins, trimmed
½ teaspoon freshly ground black pepper

Preheat oven to 500 degrees for about 15 minutes.

For the sauce, combine the vinegar, cranberries, chicken broth, sugar or honey, garlic, thyme, and onions in a medium saucepan and stir in ½ teaspoon salt. Bring to a boil. Cover, reduce heat to medium-low, and cook for 45 minutes or until the onions are almost tender, stirring occasionally. Uncover, increase the heat to medium-high, and cook for 7 minutes or until thick, stirring frequently.

Next, heat the oil in a large cast-iron skillet over medium-high heat. Sprinkle the pork evenly with the remaining salt and the pepper. Add pork to the pan and cook for 1 minute. Turn the pork over.

Place the pan in the oven and bake at 500 degrees for approximately 12 minutes (it may take up to 20-plus minutes), until a thermometer registers 155 degrees (slightly pink). Remove from the oven and let stand for 10 minutes. Slice the pork crosswise into ½-inch-thick slices. Serve with the hot cherry or cranberry sauce from the pan.

Costa Rican Sausage Tacos

I was inspired to create this dish while visiting an old and dear friend in Costa Rica. She served deliciously barbecued sausages on fresh tortillas with a bit of salsa as an appetizer. When we returned home, I adapted the idea to create a family meal that I can make year-round. It's become a favorite.

I suggest you buy the highest-quality tortillas you can find. Even the most expensive ones are relatively cheap, and a good tortilla makes a big difference. I buy the handmade ones from Trader Joe's.

Serves 4

1 tablespoon canola or other oil
1 large onion, cut into narrow strips
1 red or green bell pepper, cut into strips
Spray oil
1 package precooked chicken sausages (5 sausages)
1 can cooked black beans or homemade black beans
1 package soft corn tortillas
1 cup grated cheese of your choice (I prefer a hard Cheddar, and rather than grating it in advance, I place a hunk on the table with a grater and let everyone grate his or her own.)
Salsa to taste

OPTIONAL
Chunks of fresh avocado
Chopped lettuce
Chunks of fresh tomato

Heat a frying pan on medium heat and coat lightly with the oil. Add the onion and pepper and sauté until soft, about 10 minutes.

Heat another frying pan on medium high and coat lightly with spray oil. Place the sausages in the pan and sauté them, turning occasionally, until browned on all sides and plump.

While the onions and the sausages are cooking, heat the beans in either a saucepan or the microwave.

Close to serving time, place the tortillas on a microwave-safe plate, wrap in a clean, damp cloth, and microwave until heated through and soft. You will want to rearrange the stack (like cutting a deck of cards) partway through to ensure even heating.

Place the tortillas on the table with the salsa, cheese, and optional avocado, lettuce, and tomato, and let everyone assemble his or her own custom creation.

Acknowledgments

This project would not have been possible without the wisdom, guidance, and support of so many people. Thanks to all of you for helping me help many.

Firstly, I would like to express my deep gratitude to my agent, Yfat Reiss Gendell, for plucking me out of my hiding place and bringing me into the "book world." You were the answer to a dream I had let go of. I am ever amazed by your professionalism, competence, and responsiveness, not to mention your good taste! I feel hugely privileged to be your client. Many thanks as well to editorial assistant Cecilia Campbell-Westlind. You are a true pro at making many things happen, in very little time, in just the right way, with apparently no effort at all and an elderly dog by your side.

I would also would like to thank the foreign rights team at Foundry, Stéphanie Abou, foreign rights director, and Hannah Brown Gordon, foreign rights associate, for bringing this book to markets I hadn't even imagined. You are amazing!

Tremendous gratitude goes to my trusty cowriter, Samantha Rose, for her organization and productivity and for putting up with my endless revisions. I am truly amazed at how quickly you came up to speed on over a decade's work and study, all with grace and ease, and translated it into a truly nourishing and transformative tome. You take everything in stride, so it's easy not to notice how incredibly good you are at what you do. But I've noticed. Without you, there would be no book.

I would also like to extend my tremendous appreciation and gratitude to the incredibly capable team at Free Press. Now that I have worked with them, the huge value they add in bringing great books to the public is even clearer to me. In particular, I would like to extend my deep gratitude and respect to my editor, Leslie Meredith, for her hugely valuable feedback, calm manner, and great support through this process. You have made this a better book. I would also like to thank assistant editor Donna Loffredo for her professionalism, work ethic, and kind manner, and for making sure the process always moved smoothly. Great thanks to Dominick Anfuso, editor in chief; Martha Levin, publisher; Suzanne Donahue, associate publisher; and Laura Cooke, publishing manager. You immediately "got" the essence of this project and have supported it wholeheartedly throughout. I could not have asked for more. Again, I now know why Free Press consistently delivers top-notch titles that people want to read. Huge thanks as well to Claire Kelley and Sarah Christensen Fu for going above and beyond, pulling magical strings to make things work in the online marketing world.

Deep gratitude as well to Carisa Hays, director of publicity, for believing in this project from the beginning and putting the resources behind it to make it a success and help so many. I also want to extend a special thanks to my publicist, Jill Siegel, for truly getting this project and its potential and going the extra mile with creativity, enthusiasm, and professionalism, as well as to Nancy Inglis, my top-notch production editor, for making sure the book got where it needed to be when it needed to be there.

On a personal note, I would like to thank my husband, Stephan Fowler, for his unconditional love and support through the sometimes bumpy road that brought me here. You supported me jumping off the corporate train, with its comfy paychecks and benefits, and inventing both a new career and a new profession that I couldn't even describe in the first few years. The road got very bumpy at times, and your love only grew. You are amazing and you inspire me every day. I love you unconditionally. Much thanks as well to my loving children for inspiring me and being my teachers every day.

I would like to especially thank Susan and Tim Bratton of Personal Life Media for their maverick style, for doing things first-class, for their mentoring, and for their belief in me and support even when we brought their servers down.

Huge and deep gratitude goes to one of the finest healers of our time, my mentor, Dr. Robert Dee McDonald, for living his mission to heal the wounded heart of the world by teaching some of the most effective skills for healing, and for his openhearted support every step of the way (BTW, please write a book!). And to his wife, Dr. Luzette McDonald, who has the heart of an angel.

To the many teachers that have inspired me and helped me along the way. I offer my thanks to Connirae Andreas for her work and for working with me during her retirement. Thanks to Tim and Kris Hallbom, Steve Andreas, Gary Craig, and Robert Dilts. I have learned so much from you.

I extend my deep gratitude to my teachers, healers, and friends, especially Gina Orlando, one of the most giving, kind, compassionate, and talented professionals I know, and Hollis Polk, for your boldness in being who you are and for your talent, care, and friendship. Also, I offer great gratitude to Melinda Inn, another beautiful soul and talented healer who is boldly and gently her authentic self. I would like to offer a special acknowledgment to my colleagues who stuck with me during the storm. In particular, Stephanie Rothman, Wendi Friesen, and Mitch and Olga Stevko.

Thanks as well to my academic teachers and colleagues at the California Institute of Integral Studies, an amazing institution full of amazing people. In particular, thanks to Daniel Deslauriers, PhD, and Carol Whitfield, PhD, as well as Janis Phelps, PhD, Jorge Ferrer, PhD, Craig Chalquist, PhD, and Brendan Collins, PhD, for your gentle, loving rigor and for helping me own who I am and what I am about and take it further. Thanks also to Marina Romero, for helping me find my center that is not a center. Thanks as well to my fellow students, especially Rod Penalosa for your insightful, openhearted support. Thanks as well to Kristen Neff, PhD, for accepting my out-of-the-blue offer and for following your heart in your work.

Special thanks to my dear friend Cynthia Traina of Traina PR, who has consistently believed in me and my work and done her best pro bono efforts to help. I would also like to thank another dear friend, Samantha Miller, for her scientific input, her hot tub, and her love and humor. I must also mention my wonderful friend Anne Friscia, for her kind, courageous, and generous heart and spirit, and support every step of the way.

I would also like to thank my mother, brother, and sister-in-law for supporting me through everything and encouraging me to go for it. I love you. I also thank my dear friends Leslie Chandler and Vivian Alfonso for being with me through everything, literally and metaphorically.

I must of course thank my dedicated, competent, caring, and sweet assistant, Carrie Hayes. You have been with me through the ups and downs. I am so grateful to have you in my life. Thanks as well to my trusty webmaster, Norman Morse, for making a cozy virtual home for my many online visitors.

And I give huge thanks to my clients for being my teachers. I love you all. And special thanks to those whose stories grace these pages.

Also, I am so grateful to the members and especially to the volunteer moderators of the Inside Out Weight Loss Yahoo! group. Your generous service is such a gift to so many. Thank you.

Finally I must thank the many listeners and supporters of *Inside Out Weight Loss* who have shared their stories and gratitude with me. I also thank all the listeners I don't know for allowing me to be your guide and to do my life's work. It's awesome. Thank you for listening.

Index

Full-Filled program:
    being present in life, 122, 158
    cycle of continuous progress, 9–10,
        19–20, 242–43, 254, 269, 275
    intentions and, 12–13, 18–19
    maintaining full-filling life, 10, 269–73
    naturally slim and healthy mind-set
        and, 164, 191
    Progress Report, Week 1, 44–46
    Progress Report, Week 2, 76–77
    Progress Report, Week 3, 112–13
    Progress Report, Week 4, 161–62
    Progress Report, Week 5, 238–39
    Progress Report, Week 6, 274–75
    self-acceptance and, 149–50
    support community and, 11–15
    tools of, 3–5, 9
    underlying food issues and, 1–2
Full-Filled Weight-Release Journal:
    creating empowering beliefs, 136
    duration, intensity, frequency of
        overeating, 98, 100, 113
    Emotional Freedom Technique, 140
    exercise pros and cons, 222–23
    Feel-Good List, 85, 244–48, 274
    hunger diary, 171–79, 238
    impact of eating habits, 24
    intentions recorded in, 18–19
    limiting beliefs about weight and
        weight release, 130–31, 161
    list of "don't wants" and "do wants,"
        34–35
    list of level one self-correction tools,
        89–90, 112
    list of level three self-correction tools,
        112–13
    list of level two self-correction tools,
        90, 112
    objections recorded in, 50
    photographs in, 19, 44
    questioning old beliefs, 133–34
    small steps for exercise, 227–28
    three Ps of positive change, 253, 274
    tracking progress in, 21, 101, 116, 274
    triggers beneath the triggers, 121, 127,
        161
    use of, 10–11, 44

gratitude, 157–58, 216, 218, 245, 269, 275
guilt-neutralization strategy, 68, 80

hari hachi bu (belly eight parts), 176
helplessness, 129–30, 131
Hendricks, Gay, 177
Hicks, Esther, 260
Hicks, Jerry, 260
high-fructose corn syrup (HFCS),
    192–93, 238
Hilton, Paris, 196
holiday meals, 108–9
hopelessness, 129–30, 131
hormones, 96
hunger:
    artificial sweeteners and, 197
    cravings and, 205–6
    diary of, 171–79, 213, 238
    emotional hunger and, 170, 177
    examples of personal experiences, 175
    fears and, 167–68, 170
    managing, 207–8
    mind-set about, 164, 167–79, 187,
        188, 207, 238
    processed foods and, 194
    Re-Do and, 187–88, 189
    satisfying, 2, 3
    tuning in to, 168–70, 207
    weight release and, 172, 214
hypnotherapy, 8

inner critic:
    motivation and, 40–41
    self-acceptance and, 153–55, 159
The Inner Weigh (documentary), 4, 177
Inside Out Weight Loss audio podcast, 4, 8,
    167, 249, 271
Inside Out Weight Loss Yahoo! group,
    14, 50–51
insulin, 194–95
intentions:
    continuous improvement and, 240–
        41, 269, 275
    eating with intention, 203
    Emotional Freedom Technique and,
        140–41, 144–45, 148, 224
    forgiveness for slip-ups and, 79

identifying objections, 48
identifying what's holding you back, 115
mind-set about hunger and, 164
motivation and, 18–19, 31–32, 36–37
plateaus and, 268
positive intent of eating habits, 53–65, 68, 69, 70, 76, 95, 110, 111, 113, 121, 256
relaxed intent, 254–62
sharing, 12–13
internal tug-of-war:
    breaking overeating cycle, 66–69
    examples of personal experiences, 54–55, 62–63, 68–69, 74–75
    objections and, 48–53
    positive intent and, 53–65, 68, 69, 70
    resolving, 47, 69–75, 77

Japanese culture, 176
journal, *see* Full-Filled Weight-Release Journal

kaizen principle, 241, 242, 243, 244–48, 252
Katzen, Molly, 287

laughter:
    renewal and, 88
    self-limiting beliefs and, 135, 147
Law of Attraction, 255, 260
Leonard, George, 256, 257
life coaching, 8
The Life We Are Given (Leonard and Murphy), 256, 257
lunch recipes:
    brown rice, 283–84
    corn quesadilla, 281
    "prosocial" black beans and rice with salad, 282–84
    salmon salad, 280

McDonald, Robert Dee, 8, 12, 71
meals, structure in, 212–14
meditation:
    renewal and, 85, 88
    see also mindful meditations

mental snapshot, 19–20, 44
meridian points, 139, 142–43
metabolic syndrome, 195
mindful meditations:
    aligning appetite with slim and healthy, 200–201
    appetite adjuster, 177–79
    forgiveness, 110–11
    future self, 41–43
    gratitude and manifestation, 157–58
    journey of self-acceptance, 151–52
    relaxed intent, 259–60, 275
    replacing food as your best friend, 272
    resolving inner conflict, 72–73
    ritual eating, 217–18
mistakes, *see* slip-ups
motivation:
    away-from motivation, 28–30, 31, 45, 242, 244, 274
    behavioral change and, 19–24
    community and, 11–12, 44–45
    consequences of eating habits and, 25–27
    dream future, 37–41, 45–46
    examples of personal experiences, 31–32, 35–37, 39
    exercise and, 219–32
    impact of eating habits and, 24–25
    inner critic and, 40–41
    intentions and, 18–19, 31–32, 36–37
    research on, 7–8
    short-term and long-term, 38, 39, 93, 150
    towards motivation, 31–39, 45, 244, 274
    tracking progress and, 19–21
Murphy, Michael, 256, 257
music, 86
myth of arrival, 261

nature, 86
neurolinguistic programming (NLP), 8, 124
neuroscience, 8
Nicklaus, Jack, 102–3
nonattachment, 251–52, 256–57
nuts, 204

success sabotage, 129
sugar, 194–96, 238
support, *see* community

thirst, 205
three Ps of positive change:
    examples of personal experiences,
        250
    increasing, 253–54
    patience, 249, 251, 274
    persistence, 249–50, 274
    practice, 249, 251–53, 274
    weight release and, 248–54, 274
Total Quality Management (TQM)
        system, 241
trans fats, 192, 203, 238
trauma-release meditation, 169
triggers:
    fears and, 121–22, 127
    identifying, 3, 114, 117, 118–19, 161,
        169, 174, 265, 266
    triggers beneath triggers, 120–21, 127,
        161
    understanding, 116–23
    worthiness and, 120, 121
Twitter, 15

unconditional love, *see* self-acceptance
        and unconditional love
unique gifts, 159, 162, 270
unpronounceables, 191–92, 197, 202

videoconferencing, 15
visualization, 102–9

water, 205
water retention, weight-release
        measurement and, 96

weight loss:
    behavioral methods, 2–3, 4
    control and, 7, 17, 54, 74–75, 171
    enjoyment associated with, 17–18
    from inside out, 3–5
    as spiritual practice, 1
    see also weight release
weight release:
    continuous improvement and, 240–
        48, 275
    hunger scale and, 172, 214
    limiting beliefs about, 130–31
    measurement of, 96
    plateaus as gifts, 262–68
    positive connotations of, 18, 22
    relaxed intent and, 254–62, 275
    renewal and, 92
    self-correction and, 82
    three Ps of positive change, 248–54,
        274
weight struggle:
    mind-set of, 124, 206
    people affected by, 26
    releasing, 156–57, 270–72
    symptoms of, 25
Weight Watchers International, 4
Weston A. Price Foundation, 282
worthiness:
    exercise and, 224
    forgiveness and, 111
    positive intent and, 56–57, 58, 63, 64
    self-acceptance and, 149–50
    self-limiting beliefs and, 123, 126,
        129–30, 131
    triggers and, 120, 121
    weight loss and, 7

Yahoo! groups, 14

About the Author

A former food addict, Renée Stephens specializes in helping those who have struggled for years with their weight, helping them end their struggle for good and share their soul's gifts.

Her audio podcast, *Inside Out Weight Loss*, has been the top weight loss podcast on iTunes since its inception in 2007. Stephens was also a featured teacher in the film *The Inner Weigh*. As a behavioral weight loss expert, Stephens has consulted with Weight Watchers International and has run programs for Fortune 500 companies such as Whole Foods, Oracle, and Electronic Arts.

Stephens holds an MBA from the London Business School and a BA with distinction from the University of Virginia, and is a certified hypnotherapist, certified master practitioner of neurolinguistic programming, certified life coach, and certified destination coach. Previously, she had a successful career in marketing and international business, working for companies including IBM, Sun Microsystems, and the former PriceWaterhouse.